BODY F

SALVATION IN THE TECHNOLOGY OF PHYSICAL FITNESS

In the last three decades of the twentieth century, the p   t body became the ideal of modern Western societies. Images o.   , sculpted men and women are now ubiquitous on billboards and in magazines, film, television, and video. Science and popular culture are profoundly intertwined, and a host of exercising and dieting technologies now can make some bodies fit the taut, muscular ideal. Many people aspire to this ideal of physical fitness and the attractiveness, health, longevity, and personal security that it represents. But, as Brian Pronger argues, this approach transforms more than the body's functions and contours; it diminishes its transcendent power, compelling it to conform to a profoundly limited imagination of what the body can do.

Calling on critics of modern techno-scientific approaches to life, Pronger articulates a theory of science and of the body and pries open the texts and procedures that form the technology of physical fitness in order to consider what they try to produce. *Body Fascism* views technology not simply as a tool for other projects, but as a project itself, producing its own realities, which Pronger argues are ultimately nihilistic. Indeed, he finds disquieting parallels between what technology has done to the environment and what it is doing to the body. Exploring fascinating intersections between postmodern Western and Zen approaches to life, he shows how the body's energy is vulnerable to insidious forms of exploitation as well as capable of harbouring the potential for transcendence.

The broad scope of this book makes it unique in the discipline, and it will be of interest not only to scholars in the fields of physical education, social science, science, and technology, but also to those who are personally drawn to modern technologies of physical fitness.

BRIAN PRONGER is an associate professor in the Faculty of Physical Education and Health at the University of Toronto.

BRIAN PRONGER

Body Fascism: Salvation in the Technology of Physical Fitness

UNIVERSITY OF TORONTO PRESS
Toronto Buffalo London

© University of Toronto Incorporated 2002
Toronto Buffalo London
Printed in Canada

ISBN 0-8020-3646-5 (cloth)
ISBN 0-8020-8480-X (paper)

∞

Printed on acid-free paper

National Library of Canada Cataloguing in Publication

Pronger, Brian, 1953–
    Body fascism : salvation in the technology of physical fitness /
Brain Pronger.

Includes bibliographical references and index.
ISBN 0-8020-3646-5 (bound).
ISBN 0-8020-8480-X (pbk.)

1. Physical fitness – Social aspects.   2. Body, Human –
Social aspects.   I. Title.

GV342.P76 2002   306.4'83   C2002-901654-1

This book has been published with the help of a grant from the
Humanities and Social Sciences Federation of Canada, using funds provided
by the Social Sciences and Humanities Research Council of Canada.

University of Toronto Press acknowledges the financial assistance
to its publishing program of the Canada Council for the Arts and
the Ontario Arts Council.

University of Toronto Press acknowledges the financial support
for its publishing activities of the Government of Canada through
the Book Publishing Industry Development Program (BPIDP).

For Graeme Nicholson

Contents

What's a 'culture'? Look it up. 'A group of micro-organisms grown in a nutrient substance under controlled conditions.' A squirm of germs on a glass slide is all, a laboratory experiment calling itself a society. Most of us wrigglers make do with life on that slide; we even agree to feel proud of that 'culture'. Like slaves voting for slavery, or brains for lobotomy, we kneel down before the god of all moronic micro-organism and pray to be homogenised, or killed or engineered; we promise to obey.

Salman Rushdie, *The Ground Beneath Her Feet* (1999), 95

Preface

From the time I was very young, I loved physical activity, especially swimming and bicycling. I was not competitive and never raced. I just loved moving. There was an intensity in it that was very important for me. But the insight that I took in that way of life gradually eroded as I approached adolescence and started to realize that in my culture physical activity for boys is primarily about sport and competition, about building masculinity, about learning to take up space in aggressive and domineering ways. That did not appeal to me.

Because I did not want to be part of that masculine heterosexist cult, as I would now call it in retrospect, I avoided physical activity almost entirely from my early teen years until I was thirty, when I started swimming again in order to lose weight and shape my body to fit the *bouffant* body style that was emerging in Euro-American gay culture in the early 1980s. Like many other middle-class people, I joined the fitness craze and shaped my body according to my desire to embody the models of health and good looks circulating ever more widely in so many parts of Western consumer culture. Developing a more 'marketable' body afforded me power in terms of self-esteem and access to sexual experience. I found it reassuring to believe that I was living a more healthy way of life that would keep me young longer and stave off disease. Knowing that I had the self-discipline that it takes to be a highly fit person gave me considerable pride. Developing a fit body seemed to save me from many problems that ageing poses in modern Western culture. But something else happened as well – something that undermined the reassurances that getting fit seemed to bring me.

What started out as instrumental exercise – swimming in order to accumulate reassuring physical capital – in very short order turned out to be much more: a profound intrinsic experience. My sense of reality, of time, space, reason, and of sight, sound, and kinaesthesis, as well as my most solid senses of who, what, or how I was as a human being, my sense of the true origins of my life, was transformed by swimming. Everything that for almost twenty years had made me certain of the social structure of my finite life dissolved in the infinity to which moving through water brought me. Rilke's Third Duino Elegy describes what I felt was happening (Rilke 1989, 163–5). He offers a metaphor: a child letting go of the tender assurances given by its mother – assurances, I suggest, that parallel those that encourage us to stay with the solid way of life that comes from adhering to our socially constructed identities and hegemonic perceptions of reality:

Ah, where are the years when you shielded him just by placing
your slender form between him and the surging abyss?
How much you hid from him then. The room that filled with suspicion
at night: you made it harmless; and out of the refuge of your heart
you mixed a more human space with his night-space.
And you set down the lamp, not in that darkness, but in
your own nearer presence, and it glowed at him like a friend.
There wasn't a creak that your smile could not explain,
as though you had long known just when the floor would do that ...
And he listened and was soothed. So powerful was your presence
as you tenderly stood by the bed; his fate,
tall and cloaked, retreated behind the wardrobe, and his restless
future, delayed for a while, adapted to the folds of the curtain.

And he himself, as he lay there, relieved, with the sweetness
of the gentle world you had made for him dissolving beneath
his drowsy eyelids, into the foretaste of sleep – :
he *seemed* protected ... But inside: who could ward off,
who could divert, the floods of origin inside him?
Ah, there *was* no trace of caution in that sleeper; sleeping,
yes but dreaming, but flushed with what fevers: how he threw himself in.
All at once new, trembling, how he was caught up
and entangled in the spreading tendrils of inner event
already twined into patterns, into strangling undergrowth, prowling
bestial shapes. How he submitted –. Loved.
Loved his interior world, his interior wilderness,

that primal forest inside him, where among decayed treetrunks
his heart stood, light-green. Loved. Left it, went through
his own roots and out, into the powerful source
where his little birth had already been outlived. Loving,
he waded down into more ancient blood, to ravines
where Horror lay, still glutted with his fathers. And every
Terror knew him, winked at him like an accomplice.
Yes, Atrocity smiled ... Seldom
had you smiled so tenderly, mother. How could he help
loving what smiled at him. Even before he knew you,
he had loved it, for already while you carried him inside you, it
was dissolved in the water that makes the embryo weightless.

At the same time as my exercise was giving me assurance that I was okay, that I could fit into a youth-centred and disciplined, bourgeois, white, and able-bodied culture, it also introduced me to an alternative, infinite reality that is both terror and friend. It shook me from 'the folds of the curtain' that the cult of physical fitness was drawing. In my early thirties, swimming, running, cycling, and many other kinds of physical activity rattled me and drew me into the 'spreading tendrils of inner event,' the freedom of infinity, that the puissant moving body can produce: 'Loved. Left it, went through his own roots and out, into the powerful source where his little birth had already been outlived ...' I wanted to learn more about the body and what was possible. How does one deepen one's understanding? Where are the wise teachers – the people who can help students of the body negotiate the 'powerful source,' the 'floods of origin,' the 'primal forest,' the 'ancient blood,' the smiles of 'atrocity'? Where does one turn to learn the wisdom of the moving body? How does one learn to teach that wisdom? How does one go about devoting one's life to this goal?

I thought that the path might lead through physical education. And so I took my aquatic rediscovery of the body, dropped my career as a violinist and teacher, and returned to university to study physical education. Modern physical education, it turned out, casts wisdom primarily as the technology of physical fitness, which understands the body as a biophysical object whose functions can be maximized by instrumental programs of training and diet. The technological vision of the body and of exercise dominates physical education, government policies on health and fitness, and the physical fitness industry. I found that the technological approach to the body overshadowed the more Rilkean insights that I was beginning to develop. With this book I explore what in that techno-scientific approach I find troubling.

The technology of physical fitness is a discourse of texts, socio-cultural practices, and bodily procedures that produce human life in controlled ways: increased physical control in terms of muscular strength, endurance, and flexibility, and greater cardio-vascular efficiency for the sake of better athletic performance or greater control over health in terms of disease prevention, both physical and mental – living longer and more efficiently, for instance. The technology also plays a growing role in sculpting the body for a fashionable look – typically lean, muscular, and youthful. These objectives often intertwine, with some being more important at times than others. So, for instance, a person interested primarily in attaining a lean, visibly muscular body will focus on muscle-building exercises and will do some cardio-vascular work in order to burn fat; better cardio-vascular functioning may be a by-product of this focus, and so may improved overall health. If the person is striving for an extremely muscular look, he or she may do little or no cardio-vascular exercise and may reduce fat by using diet and drug supplements – in which case, the technology of physical fitness interferes with good health, increasing a person's vulnerability to various diseases, such as liver failure, heart disease, and anorexia nervosa. Similarly, someone may be interested in physical fitness 'purely' for 'health' reasons. To avoid heart disease or osteoporosis, a woman may take up a program of walking, jogging, running, or cycling; reduced fat and greater strength could be a by-product of this focus. Or a competitive athlete may be interested in furthering a professional career as a hockey player and, depending on the position that she or he plays, engage in an exercise and dietary program that builds the requisite physical capacities; long-term health in professional sports is often completely unrelated to, if not undermined by, sport-specific training (Hoberman 1992). There are also health-based programs of physical fitness that try to balance all the components. While the specific goals and efficacies of particular technologies of physical fitness vary considerably, the technology as a whole shares a common approach to the body, a common philosophy of what the body is and can be. It is this common philosophy of the body in the technology of physical fitness that I analyse in this book.

As I said above, the technology of physical fitness is a discourse of texts, socio-cultural practices, and bodily procedures that produce the body. The texts of this technology – analysed in chapter 3 below – include scholarly scientific papers on the physiology and psychology of physical fitness; academic textbooks on the sciences of physical fitness; manuals for exercise and dietary regimes; and popular books on physical fitness, as well as magazines and audio and video tapes dedicated to physical fitness and body building. By virtue of their contribution to popular conceptions of the body, other magazines, books, films, and videos that feature the 'fit body' also serve as texts of the technology of physical fitness, including fashion magazines for men and women, soft- and hard-core pornographic videos and magazines, cyborg movies such as Arnold Schwarzenegger's *Terminator* movies, and the American television series *Baywatch* on beach patrols. This is not to say that there are not important differences in the shapes of the bodies in these various representations, differences represented by race, gender, class, (dis)ability, and the changing fashions for leanness and muscularity in consumer culture. But as I argue in chapter 3, they represent a common underlying philosophy of the body that the differences do not significantly change.

The texts do not exist independently of one another. They constitute what Julia Kristeva (1980) calls an intertextual ensemble, both reflecting and producing the socio-historical contexts in which they operate. For instance, the popular image of the lean, muscular body textually rendered in fashion magazines reflects the scientific texts on the physiology of exercise and muscular development; these bodies are the products of scientific knowledge. Similarly, the socio-cultural desirability of the lean, muscular body informs scientific research as the object that the technology of physical fitness can produce; the development of commercial products and the hope for resulting financial profit funds scientific research on, for example, exercise machines and running shoes. I explore the relationship between scientific textuality and social context more deeply in chapter 1.

The socio-cultural practices of this technology are often at work in government policies and initiatives on physical fitness; in physical education in schools; in professional, elite, amateur, masters', age-group, and recreational sports; and in the physical fitness industry (fitness and sports clubs, fitness classes, personal training businesses, fitness equipment businesses, sports clothing businesses, and so on). Technological body procedures are at work in physical fitness testing, high-performance athletic training, popular workout routines, and dietary and lifestyle regimens, as well as in therapeutic exercises for the damaged or disabled body. We can 'read' all of these texts, socio-cultural practices, and body procedures for their technological imperatives, for the ways in which they understand and go about producing the body.

Acknowledgments

This book was made possible by grants from the Canada Council for the Arts, the Connaught Foundation, the Ontario Arts Council, and the Social Sciences and Humanities Research Council of Canada. Because it is a highly intertextual work, I owe an enormous debt to the many writers cited or alluded to. I have benefited immensely from a circle of friends with whom I have discussed these ideas over the years. I give many thanks in particular to my wonderful teacher and friend, Graeme Nicholson, to whom I dedicate the book. I also fondly acknowledge the contributions of the members of my swimming-and-Heidegger-reading group, which we called the Dasein Swim Club – Jay Cassell, Peter Ellinger, Trish Glazebrook, and Gerry Oxford – as well as those of Fadi Abou-Rihan and my dear friend Jim Bartley. The support of my dean, Bruce Kidd, and other colleagues at the University of Toronto has been invaluable. I am grateful for the support and enthusiasm of my editor at the University of Toronto Press, Virgil Duff, as well as for the thoughtful and careful copy editing of John Parry.

BODY FASCISM:
SALVATION IN THE TECHNOLOGY OF PHYSICAL FITNESS

Introduction: Reading the Science and Technology of Physical Fitness

What is it we are a part of that we do not see?
Loren Eisely, cited in Martin 1999, 193

In the last three decades of the twentieth century the physically fit body became the ideal, if not always the reality, of modern Western societies. Images of the lean, sculpted body are now ubiquitous in the popular representations of magazines, billboards, film, television, and video. Popular books on physical fitness and diet have become a significant presence in most bookstores and one of the most successful sellers on the internet. Even small towns boasted fitness clubs and facilities in their community centres. And physical fitness products for the home now constitute a multi-billion-dollar industry in North America. But physical fitness has become not only a phenomenon of popular culture. The governments of most industrial and post-industrial countries now actively promote programs and support scientific research to develop the fitness of their populations. There is a substantial academic scientific literature on physical fitness. Physical fitness has become the centrepiece of physical education for children, adults, and the elderly. And the scientific technology of physical fitness has become the intellectual and applied foundation of universities' physical education departments, most of which are now called departments of 'kinesiology.' As Haraway, Aronowitz, and others have argued, science and popular culture are profoundly mixed in the contemporary scene. I argue in chapter 3 that this is particularly the case in the technology of physical fitness.

Building on the scholarly literature that has been critical of the cults and industries of physical fitness, this book deconstructs the phenomenon as a modernist technological approach to life. Drawing particularly on the work of Heidegger, Deleuze and Guattari, and Foucault, and examining intersections between postmodern Western and Eastern (particularly Zen Buddhist) approaches to life, it develops a theory of the body and of science and technology that analyses the nature of desire in modernity as it is manifest in the techno-culture of physical fitness.

The dominant understanding of the technology of physical fitness, both popularly and in most academic discourse, is that it is a practical way to maximize the body's natural physiological and psychological capacity. Taking advantage of modern scientific knowledge of the body (exercise physiology, nutrition, and biomechanics) and of the mind (exercise psychology), this technology is the most modern approach to physical and mental performance. Not all the techniques have the same academic scientific credibility – it is commonplace among professional physical educators to deride the unscientific 'quacks' who are part of the physical fitness industry (Mrozek 1987). For that reason there are various 'credentiallizing' professional governing bodies, such as the American College of Sports Medicine (ACSM), and the Canadian Society for Exercise Physiology (CSEP), that attempt to ground their particular approach to physical fitness in modern exercise sciences. Fraudulence and quackery aside, the dominant understanding of the technology is that it provides one of the best ways to live life most productively and to the fullest. Certainly, there are many debates about what particular technological approaches are the most effective – for instance, debates about what intensity of aerobic exercise is optimal for the best training effect, about the wisdom of drug supplements, about which fats are unhealthy, about what exercises produce the most effective results, and about the most effective timing for stretching. But there has been insufficient concern in physical education – understood broadly as physical education in schools, recreational and high-performance sport, and the physical fitness industry – about the techno-scientific approach to the body as such.

Over the last two decades, a scholarly literature, critical of the cultures of physical fitness, has developed. While the social sciences and humanities have been significantly marginalized in the academic discourses of physical education – overtaken by science and technology – they have not been totally silenced. There is a valuable, albeit small, socio-cultural literature critical of dominant policies and models of the techno-scientific approach to the body. It pursues a number of themes. It analyses the ways in which the technology has developed in relation to the problems of the welfare state and capitalist individualism.[1] Gender has been an important axis – the literature has criticized the technology of physical fitness as a cultural practice for the production of gender difference. These practices have contributed to the polarization and hierarchialization of the genders,[2] the marginalization of people who do not fit those polar distinctions or who challenge the hierarchies,[3] the production of gendered power by physical strength or weakness that works to 'naturalize' power difference,[4] and a virtual epidemic of exercise and eating disorders produced by the tyranny of changing images of the ideally fit body.[5]

The gender critiques unanimously maintain that gender differences emerge not only between the sexes, but also within them.[6] Some critics of physical fitness have analysed it as a 'technology' of social discipline.[7] This analysis emanates from the work of Michel Foucault, who is pivotal to recent histories of the body in modernity. In this framework, the services of health and wellness professionals, rather than rediscovering and restoring the body, have been instrumental in harnessing its energies in the production of social control. Scientific knowledge and the scientization of physical education have been centred in the production of this social control, an issue that I pursue at length in chapter 1.[8] Also, out of feminist critiques of paradigmatic biases in scientific research there have developed critiques of ageist, sexist, racist, and ethnocentric biases in the exercise sciences. Other commentators have criticized the scientization of physical education for the way it aids the establishment of professional hegemonies (Beamish 1982; Harvey 1986; MacIntosh and Whitson 1990; McKay, Gore, and Kirk 1990; Whitson and MacIntosh 1990), for its rationalization and mechanization of the body (Harvey 1986; McKay, Gore, and Kirk 1990), as well for its technocentric (Bain 1990; Charles 1998) or technocratic (McKay, Gore, and Kirk 1990) ideology.

Critics of physical fitness have overlooked an interesting body of writing in philosophy, history, anthropology, and sociology of science. Those authors who have appealed to Foucault's theoretical frameworks have made mention of his philosophy and history of scientific knowledge, but only in passing, and they do not plumb his analysis of the intimate connection between power and scientific knowledge.[9] All the writers who have been critical of the scientization of physical edu-

cation have been so because they see in it negative political consequences. Yet they do not directly address the literature from the philosophy and sociology of science that could explain the powerful politics of scientific knowledge – the way in which scientific knowledge
shapes the world in which we live. The materialist critiques of the
scientific professionalization of physical education, describing the development of professional monopolies, come closest to an account of
the power of science. But they go no further than citing the high status
of science as a guarantor of legitimacy. As I argue in the chapter 1,
there is more to the prestige of science than mere status: science is
prestigious because it is so effective at changing the world. The power
of the exercise sciences needs to be analysed for the ways in which
they set out to change the reality of the body. Most of the critics of the
science of the technology of physical fitness, while they do not have
explicit theories of scientific knowledge, suggest implicitly that the
sciences are problematic because their *ideas* of the nature of the human
body and of the politics that contribute to its health or disease are
inappropriate: the exercise sciences convey *false ideologies*, which is to
say that their ideas about the body (understood, for example, metaphorically as a machine) and of health (as a primarily individual concern) are at odds with the *true* nature of the body and strategies for
health. There is a stronger, indeed in some senses more material, critique of the exercise sciences, which argues that they are problematic
not because of their *ideas* about the body and its politics, but because
of the way in which they attempt to actually *produce* the body and its
politics. I pursue this political philosophy of science in chapter 1.

It is also notable that, except for Vertinsky and Harvey, few critics
have examined the actual texts of exercise science. While Vertinsky's
analyses are prescient and offer excellent historical treatments of racist, sexist, and ageist ideologies in science, they, like the rest of the
critical literature, ignore the substantial critical scholarship that has
developed over the last thirty years or more in the sociology, philosophy, and history of science and scientific textuality. Those authors
who invoke Foucault's analysis of the body and social organization do
not appeal to his companion analysis of the sciences of the body. This
leaves the bulk of the literature critiquing only the *application* of scientific knowledge of physical fitness, not the *knowledge* itself. Proponents
of the sciences of physical fitness can then argue that their research is
sound and that the problem lies outside the proper realm of science
and instead in politics, policy, and so on. A stronger critique, which I

attempt to develop in the next chapters, suggests that the fundamental orientation of the exercise sciences is problematic.

Those authors who have engaged recent French social theory, namely in the work of Foucault and Bourdieu, have touched on the ways in which the body is a site for socio-cultural discourse. While Foucault and Bourdieu are obviously indispensable to any analysis of the body in modernity, there has been a flourishing of critical, reflective work on the body in social theory that enhances and reaches beyond them and that the literature on physical fitness overlooks. A fully-fledged theory of the body, in the light of recent continental European per-spectives, has yet to be developed and applied to the cult of physical fitness. McKay (McKay, Gore, and Kirk 1990) comments: 'One would imagine that a field calling itself human movement studies/science, human kinetics, kinesiology, kinanthropology, or physical education (especially when its professional leaders so frequently point to its al-leged links with Greek culture and its sound mind/sound body pre-supposition) would have sophisticated discourses about human bod-ies. Although anthropologists, historians, philosophers, sociologists, and feminists have produced an impressive amount of literature about what Fay (Fay 1987) has called somatic knowledge, it is mainly a few cultural historians, sociologists, feminists, and maverick physical edu-cators who are aware of its implications for physical education' (59).

The literature that has engaged continental European perspectives on the body has done so primarily in a negative fashion: the body as a site of oppression and subjugation to discourse. There is no definition of the body in the critical literature on physical fitness. While there has been considerable discussion of the abuses of the body in society, as a machine, as gendered, raced, classed, and so on, there has been no consideration of what in the body's nature makes it possible to be mechanized, gendered, raced, and classed. That is to say, there has been no attention to the ways in which the body is open to discursive appropriation, to the power of the body to be 'discoursed.' The posi-tive power of the body to engage or resist discourse needs to be con-sidered. Moreover, the erotic body, or desire, is mostly absent in the socio-cultural literature on physical fitness. As Caroline Fusco (in progress) points out, discussions of desire have been limited to ques-tions of sexuality, and even there fairly simplistically, in binaries of homo- and hetero- sexualities.

A couple of authors mention the pleasures of physical activity and the fact that it has been left out of most technologies of physical fitness, especially out of science-based physical education (Featherstone 1991; McKay, Gore, and Kirk 1990), but they do so only in passing, in a couple of sentences. Pleasure or desire is not central to any discussions of physical education, except negatively, where physical education is constructed as strategic in the control of desire (the desire to indulge in delicious, fattening foods, for example). A positive sense of the body's pleasure and desire could make a positive contribution. In short, a thorough theory of the body has yet to be offered. Except for some discussion of Foucault on the body (Bordo 1993; Featherstone 1991; Harvey 1986; Harvey and Sparks 1991; Kirk and Spiller 1994; Kirk and Tinning 1994; Kirk and Twigg 1994; Kirk 1994; McKay, Gore, and Kirk 1990), there are no explicit theories of the body in the literature. And, most important, there is little theorizing on the horizons of transcendence in modern body culture.

I argue in chapter 2 that any adequate theory of the body and subsequent analysis of it in modern society, especially in physical education, broadly defined, requires an appreciation of the body's erotic power. I suggest that only with an appreciation of that very power is it possible to imagine a *physical* education that sets its sights on freedom, rather than on subjugation.

In this chapter on method, I first explain how I propose to analyse the technology of physical fitness and, second, describe the intertextual relation between this book and the authors whom it engages.

The Philosophy of the Limit

This section describes how I analyse the technology of physical fitness. It outlines a type of inquiry that looks at the ways in which various systems impose limits on reality, thus producing particular realities, and it suggests ways of thinking about dimensions that are left out of systems, such as the technology of physical fitness. Drucilla Cornell calls it the 'philosophy of the limit,' and it brings us to the powerful concepts of secondness and of alterity, or otherness.

A naturalistic reading of the technology of physical fitness seems simple and straightforward enough: scientific technologies of the body have penetrated its inner workings, have come closer than any earlier knowledge to understanding its functions and consequently have developed an array of techniques for maximizing its potential. If people order their lives in accordance with the technology of physical fitness, they will live longer, be healthier, and ultimately enjoy greater freedom and a more satisfying life than those who do not. In short, the technology of physical fitness represents a practical, *modern* way of living life to the fullest. But I argue that this modern approach to amplifying life's natural possibilities also limits it.

Over the last thirty years the naturalness of Nature has been the subject of considerable critique. Regarding the body, this critique has emanated from political activists who contest the ways in which bodies have been negatively represented by the dominant discourses of the natural body: women, people of colour, sexual minorities, people with disabilities, people of the so-called third world, and so on. Feminists have criticized the 'natural inferiority' of women and 'natural superiority' of men; anti-racists, the 'natural differences' of race; homosexuals, the 'unnaturalness' of their sexual desires and the 'natural superiority' of heterosexuality; people with disabilities, the 'natural incapacity' of their bodies; and 'third world peoples,' the 'primitiveness' of their desire. These differences have been scrutinized for being socially constructed systems of domination that are perpetuated under the guise of being 'natural.' Questioning 'nature' is key to postmodern criticism. Linda Hutcheon (1989) says: 'The postmodern's initial concern is to de-naturalize some of the dominant features of our way of life, to point out that those entities that we unthinkingly experience as "natural" (they might even include capitalism, patriarchy, liberal humanism) are in fact "cultural"; made by us, not given to us. Even nature, postmodernism might point out, doesn't grow on trees' (2).

A few words on 'postmodernism' are in order here. Debates on modernity and postmodernity continue to rage. Is modernity finished (Habermas 1983)? Is modernity killing us (Levin 1987)? Are we in a postmodern era (Huyssen 1986; Jameson 1984; Latour 1993; Lyotard 1984; Readings and Schaber 1993; Smart 1990)? Is postmodernism intellectually sound (Dews 1987; Lash 1990, 1996; Rosenthal 1992; Turner 1990)? Is postmodernism a viable political framework (Callari, Cullenberg, and Biewener 1995; Doan 1994; Ebert 1996; Grossberg 1992; Phelan 1994)? Since it would be inappropriate to get into the complexities of those debates here, I say simply that I sympathize with much of the critical impetus that is often signified by the term 'postmodern.' And as the rest of this book shows, I draw extensively from the work of writers who are in one way or another considered 'postmodern.' I do not want to constrain the following analysis to any particular postmodern 'orthodoxy,' if such a thing were even possible from a postmodern perspective. I do, however, want to align my analysis with the broad intellectual, political, and ultimately 'spiritual' commitments that I believe are characteristic of most postmodern perspectives. Linda Hutcheon (1989) has summarized those commitments, saying they always involve five elements:

- critiques of domination
- awareness that dominating 'power is not something unitary that exists outside us' (3)
- awareness that dominating power lurks in what are often the most seemingly benign texts
- awareness of the critic's inevitable complicity in the very power structures being criticized
- the consequent obligation to self-reflexivity

Postmodern political activists, then, are keenly aware of the complex ways in which their political critiques and projects are intimately tied to, indeed complicitous in, the very sources of domination that they would try to resist, transgress, subvert, or transform. Hutcheon qualifies this, saying: 'But complicity is not full affirmation or strict adherence; the awareness of difference and contradiction, of *being inside and outside*, is never lost in the feminist, as in the postmodern' (Hutcheon 1989, 14, emphasis added). While the forms of dominating power critiqued by feminist, queer, anti-racist, environmentalist, and other activists may be insidious,[10] the grasp of such power is not necessarily total. And that grasp is weakened by sensitivity to the myriad ways in which power hides itself. Heightened sensitivity to the paradoxical intimacy that domination and critical resistance find in each other characterizes the work of most of the writers that I invoke for the rest of this book. As Drucilla Cornell (1992) points out, 'Humility before the paradox undermines the self-righteousness that Nietzsche so despised' (90).

Identifying the insidious operations of dominating power has become crucial to many political activists and scholars. My analysis of the technology of physical fitness joins that endeavour. Methodologically, this is an examination of the ways in which the technology of physical fitness constitutes a *discourse* on the body that seeks to foreclose on its potential, disguising itself as a way of doing precisely the opposite. Drawing on Foucault, Toby Miller (1993) suggests that discourse be 'understood not as a universe of meaning but as a complex that combines "the action of imposed scarcity, with a fundamental power of affirmation"' (Foucault 1981, 73). I attempt to show the ways in which the technology of physical fitness constitutes a complex of statements and practices of the body that limits its potential by affirming particular modes of being. In so doing, this discourse of physical fitness sets out to 'determine actions and thoughts ... [It] is a particular grammar that permits the making of choices only within its own rules. It decides what can and cannot be said, done, or represented' (Miller 1993, xiv). Robert Barsky (1993, 35) says: 'Discourse analysis theory proposes that relations of power in our society affect and shape the way we both communicate with each other and create "knowledge."' As Foucault (1979, 27) writes: 'There is no power relation without the correlative constitution of a field of knowledge, nor any knowledge that does not presuppose and constitute at the same time power relations.' The task, therefore, of my analysis is to reveal the ways in which power secrets itself discursively in the seemingly apolitical technology of physical fitness. It is crucial to keep in mind that a discourse, like a conversation, does not simply impose a reality, one-sidedly. It can never be a *fait accompli*; it is an active, ongoing process that productively coerces life, engaging it precisely in the complex tension between resistance and compliance.

I draw my analysis from the critical path that the postmodern feminist legal scholar Drucilla Cornell has called the 'the philosophy of the limit.' I argue that this type of analysis is particularly adept at revealing the hidden and oppressive operations of power in everyday discourses, such as the technology of physical fitness. 'The philosophy of the limit' has traditionally gone by the name 'deconstruction,' about which there has been considerable scholarly and political debate (Critchley 1992; Dews 1987; Morrison 1996; Silverman 1989). A frequent critique of deconstruction has been that it is preoccupied with taking apart the play of language, sliding into a ludic idealism that is not only politically futile but also ethically suspect, preferring elitist intellectual games to concrete political action. Deconstruction, it is claimed, fails to 'grasp' material reality, the 'real' lives of people who suffer from the material organization of life that perpetuates privilege in the contexts of class, race, gender, sexuality, ethnicity, and so on, realities that some claim are best understood by 'materialist' critiques (for example, Ebert 1996; Messner 1996; Morton 1996).

Cornell has argued that so-called materialist arguments against deconstruction fail to appreciate the subtlety and political commitment of its approach, which she says is concerned essentially with exposing the ways in which seemingly innocuous, indeed well-intentioned systems do violence, both symbolically and 'materially,' to our potential for living full lives. Jacques Derrida (1978), among the most influential practitioners of deconstruction, says that all systems (which would include linguistic, artistic, social, athletic, sexual, scientific, or technological) impose structural limits on the power to appreciate material reality. Such limits preclude our engaging in fully and genuinely ethical relationships with material reality, which in turn undermines our political power to formulate alternative constructions of reality. The point of deconstruction is to expose the insensitivity to the power of limitation that lurks within a system and to show that this insensitivity prevents our having ethical relationships with any body or any thing that is other – other either to the *operators* of the system or to the *system itself.* Deconstruction seeks to reveal what is left out and to show how such exclusions prohibit just, ethical relations. A deconstruction of the technology of physical fitness, therefore, would try to expose what that technology leaves out and what that marginalization indicates about the political program of the discourse.

Deconstruction, by the seeming negativity of the word itself, is sometimes confused with a kind of cynical, nihilistic reductionism – take apart the constructs and you are left with nothing. Some sociologists, philosophers, and political activists, thinking that deconstruction reduces everything to a cynical and unreconstructable litter, believe that it renders political action impossible (Dews 1987; Ebert 1996; Habermas 1983). To counteract such misunderstanding, Cornell (1992) has suggested renaming the project 'the philosophy of the limit.' Questioning limits has been central to the work of the activist movements that I mentioned above: feminists questioning the limits of gender, anti-racists, the limits of racism, and postmodernists, the limits of modernity (Game 1991; Gray 1995; Hutcheon 1989; Jameson 1984; Lyotard 1984; Miller 1993); the handicapped, the limits of ablism, gays, the limits of homophobia and heterosexism, and queers, the limits of gay culture (Champagne 1995; Kipnis 1993; Warner 1993); and post-queers, the limits of queer (Simpson 1996). All these scholars have engaged in some philosophy of the limit, questioning the ways in which social, economic, cultural, and bodily systems construct the limits of human possibilities. Clearly, there are activist political agendas in them all. Simply put: what limits are operative? how can they be justified? and where and how might it be wise to dismantle them?

Deconstruction in Derrida's method interrogates the limits of systems as such. While there is much to this metacritique, a brief discussion of three elements raised by Cornell as concerns of the philosophy of the limit should suffice for this chapter: 'the logics of parergonality,' 'secondness,' and 'alterity.'

Derrida (1987) coined the expression 'the logics of parergonality' to name the way in which the establishment of any system as a system suggests a beyond to it. That beyond consists of that which the system excludes, by virtue either of what it cannot comprehend or of what it prohibits in order to accomplish its systematic objectives. The philosophy of the limit asks about what lies beyond a particular system by virtue of its existence as a system and what the system's limits are. How do the science and technology of physical fitness form a coherent system for producing the body? What elements of the body do they leave out of the system? What kind of body do they produce, given that they exclude dimensions of it? How does the technology of physical fitness make the body fit the limitations of wider discourses that are circulating in the particular historical context?

The word 'parergon' is a compound of the Greek *para*, meaning 'alongside' or 'subsidiary,' and *ergon*, meaning work, and it refers therefore to the by-product of a larger work (*Shorter Oxford Dictionary*, 1993). Both the work, *ergon*, and the by-product, *para*, are 'at work' in the logic of parergonality. Therefore we need to examine the logics of parergonality, both for what they exclude and for what they include; for together these produce the ultimate work of a particular system. Several questions constitute my undertaking here. What is at work in the technology of physical fitness? What is its *ergon*? What is its *para*? What kind of life do the logics of parergonality attempt to produce? What limits are effected? How is human potential rendered selectively concrete in the technology of physical fitness? To what end?

The philosophy of the limit, looking at parergonality, asks what it leaves out, what it makes other, excludes, rejects. What by-products does a system produce? The corollary of this asks: when something is left out, what is produced by virtue of what is left in? How does exclusion affect that which is included? How does the excluded, by virtue of its exclusion, produce the particular reality of that which is included?

The problem of parergonality may not be just the problem of exclusion – i.e., it excludes some people or some dimensions of life from the benefits of the system; it may also be a problem of subtraction. The limits imposed by parergonality, by their power of *exclusion*, may also diminish that which the system *includes*. In other words, that which it includes and the reality that results may be diminished, indeed transformed, by its alienation from what it excludes.

A simple – and admittedly reductionist – observation may serve as an example. A patriarchal political system, such as the prevalent system of electoral politics, includes men and for the most part excludes women – consider the gender balance of the Canadian House of Commons. The problem is not only that women are mostly absent from the House, with men reaping the full benefits of inclusion, and women not. The problem is also that the absence of women diminishes the House, as does the exclusive inclusion of men. In short, there is a less-than-full concretization of human potential in exclusively male political systems. The logic of parergonality at work in patriarchal electoral politics diminishes the potential of the politics by rendering possibilities selectively concrete.

Describing the philosophy of the limit, Cornell (1992) also draws on what C.S. Peirce, in his critique of Hegelian idealism, called 'secondness' – 'the materiality that persists *beyond* any attempt to conceptualize it. Secondness, in other words, is what resists. Very simply, reality is not interpretation all the way down' (1). The philosophy of the limit asks about what realities resist and persist beyond systems of interpretation. It inquires about that which the system makes other. The technology of physical fitness, as a systematic method of producing life, of realizing the body, is also a system of interpreting the body, of interpreting life, of representing what the body is and can be. What realities of the body do the scientific conception and the technological reproduction of it make other? What do they render second to the technologically produced body? How does that which is rendered other in this technology resist the technology? To what extent is the reality of the body that is rendered second by the technology of physical fitness inaccessible to those who have embodied the technology? To what extent do modern technological modes of existence render these realities invisible? Do they render these realities so secondary to dominant technological modes of existence that they are for the most part incomprehensible, or even virtually nonexistent? Have the modern technologies of the body been so successful in producing bodies, in representing visions of what the body is, that there seems to be nothing else? In short, can a conceptual and reproductive system such as the modern technology of the body be so effective in shaping the modern imagination of the body that the resulting 'secondary,' other dimensions disappear without a trace? What kind of life is left?

In the Preface I wrote about the 'powerful source,' the wonder and infinity that I discovered in swimming. And I said that when I started to study physical education, that dimension was completely absent from everything that we were taught. The technological education that I was receiving rendered the wonder second. And as I survey the array of scientific, government, and commercial texts on physical fitness, I hear only silence in this regard. The technology of physical seems deaf to this dimension of life. So the question of secondness here is: what kind of life is produced in such deafness? But another question also arises: what latent possibilities does that silence hold?

Cornell suggests exploring secondness, exploring that which is made to disappear, via Theodor Adorno's technique of negative dialectics. Negative dialectics attempts to discover difference *in* identity. It attempts to reveal negatively what a concept, a system, a technology leaves out, not by appropriating it conceptually, not by including it within the very system that effects its erasure, but by knowing it indirectly precisely as that which the system omits. Adorno says that this is not a transcendental method or reality, for that would reify it also as a concept. 'Negative dialectics is instead the "truth" of an *unreconciled* reality, or antagonistic entirety, to be found in "the cognitive confrontation of concept and thing"' (Cornell 1992, 20, emphasis added). So by coming into a *dialectical* relation with what a system includes, we can come to negative knowledge of what it leaves out. This is decidedly not the same as bringing in what it omits. The excluded remains outside, unviolated by the system of knowledge. Negative dialectics is the opposite of the power-knowledge that Foucault has identified with the conquering gaze of science and technology (Foucault 1975). 'Regarding the concrete utopian possibility, dialectics is the ontology of the wrong state of things. The right state of things would be free of it' (Adorno 1973, 11).

But because utopia is far from us, we need alternative strategies. The philosophy of the limit attempts to detect what the logics of parergonality renders second without violating the 'freedom' that exclusion from the system ironically accords secondness. In this study of the technology of physical fitness, my analytical task becomes one of exposing what of the body the technological system excludes without harnessing its freedom – i.e., knowing it negatively. My quest here is to remain faithful to the body's materialism, in the sense that Adorno means materialism – i.e., engaging in the negative dialectics that permits identification (which Adorno calls 'mimesis') with that which dominant discourses of the body have made other, without incorporating it into an epistemic system – i.e., without making it functional within a system's economy, by allowing it to remain free of the system. There is an emotional dimension to negative dialectics, a sense of longing for that which is lost but not entirely forgotten. This is why Adorno calls such work a 'melancholy science.'

Adorno's melancholy science 'speaks to us now because his implicit ethical vision rests on expansiveness rather than on constriction' (Cornell 1992, 37). I hope to show that the expansiveness implicit in the longing for that which dominant discourses may systematically remove can be particularly useful for seeing the philosophy of the limit in the technology of physical fitness. Adorno's expansive imagination reminds us that there can be more to life than what has come to pass in dominant discourses. Just as Heidegger's analysis of the *das Man* mode of everyday existence suggests that more is possible where there is deep suspicion about the fulness of everyday modes of being, so too Adorno's melancholy invites transcendence. 'The presentation of the "more-than-this" serves as a corrective to realist and conventionalist ethics with their shared impulse to enclose us in our form of life,' which, Cornell (1992) suggests, is profoundly shaped by 'the ideology of lesser expectations' (17). Adorno's 'is a gentle, directive message,' whose melancholy focuses 'on the development of an attitude of tenderness toward otherness and gentleness towards oneself as a sensual creature' (37).

The philosophy of the limit must therefore approach with great care its object – the fulness of the body, including its 'other' dimensions, which are beyond its technological limits. Those elements of life, of the body, that the science and technology of physical fitness most profoundly excludes are probably the most delicate dimensions, the most vulnerable to violation by the prying eyes of science, including this study. The ethics of the philosophy of the limit, Cornell argues, must be the ethics of alterity. 'Alterity' refers to an ethical philosophy that remains open, indeed committed, to fostering the ways in which the other is differentiated from and inaccessible to systems of interpretation and social organization. Derrida says that for the other to be appreciated of itself, it must remain other to the system. 'For Derrida, the excess to the system cannot be known positively [by the system] ...

We must try, if we are to remain faithful to the ethical relationship, to heed [the other's] otherness to any system of conventional definition' (Cornell 1992, 2).

Cornell grounds the philosophy of the limit in the ambitious ethical quest to engage the other and otherness non-violently: 'The entire project of the philosophy of the limit is driven by the ethical desire to enact the ethical relation ... the aspiration to a nonviolent relationship to the Other and to otherness more generally, that assumes responsibility to guard the Other, against the appropriation that would deny her [its] difference and singularity' (2). The ethics of inclusion, which tries to bring otherness into a system while requiring it to manifest itself within the structure of the system, appropriates otherness, making it conform to the system.[11] The ethics of alterity, in contrast, works not by inclusion but by openness – openness to otherness in a way that allows the other to deconstruct the system, to call into question the system's limits, particularly in its appropriation of others' otherness. Alterity in this study entails an analysis of the ways in which the technology remains open to or forecloses on the fulness of the body. In what ways does the technology of physical fitness appreciate that which is other to it? Asking the question of alterity also necessitates taking great care to ensure that it enter into a non-violent relationship to the body, that it guard the body's elusive otherness and not inadvertently repeat an appropriating parergonal logic. That is the postmodern commitment to self-reflexivity that I mentioned above.

As we contemplate the other of the technology of physical fitness, to which I have alluded as the 'powerful source' – the wonder and infinity that I began to discover in my experience of physical activity but realized was lacking in the technology – we need to be very careful that we not rein in its power, appropriating its otherness into yet another system.

The philosophy of the limit does not suggest some simple eradication of limits. Life, of course, would be impossible if there were no limits. The traditional etymological definition of philosophy is that it is the love of wisdom. The philosophy of the limit is the love of wisdom about limits. What are wise ways of constructing limits? How can limits be constructed with an ethics of alterity? So my ethical question becomes: what wisdom is there in the ways that the interpretations and organization of the technology of physical fitness limit or foster the potentialities for difference and otherness in the body?

The philosophy of the limit, being concerned essentially with questions of difference and otherness, enters into some of the most crucial issues of politics, philosophy, and human relations. Mark Taylor (1987) begins his study of identity and difference, entitled *Altarity*, saying: 'The history of society and culture is, in large measure, a history of the struggle with the endlessly complex problems of difference and otherness. Never have the questions posed by difference and otherness been more pressing than they are today. For an era dominated by the struggle between, among, and against various "isms" – communism, fascism, totalitarianism, capitalism, racism, sexism, etc. – the issue of difference is undeniably political' (xxi).

This book seeks to uncover the politics of identity and difference in the science and technology of physical fitness, to expose the ways in which seemingly innocuous and well-intentioned knowledge power systems have done violence both symbolically and materially to our potential for living full and active lives. It attempts to pry open the texts that form the technology of physical fitness in order to consider critically the difference that they attempt to deny and what, in so doing, they try to produce.

What is truth in the philosophy of the limit? How are we to understand truth in the words below? In 'The Essence of Truth,' Heidegger (1961) says that the usual concept of truth involves a 'correct' correspondence between the meaning of a statement and the state of affairs that the author means it to signify, an accurate alignment of the sign and the signified. If, for instance, I say that 'there is a red book lying on my desk,' it is a true statement if there actually is such a book on my desk. Obviously such a concept is useful, especially if I am asking someone to fetch that red book from my desk. It is a useful concept where there is social agreement – that is, a traditional acceptance of the commensurability between certain signifying practices and signified realities. However, where there are attempts to speak about realities that lie well outside traditional agreements about what constitutes particular realities and what signs adequately refer to them, a correspondence theory of truth is inadequate to the task. This problem is most palpable when we pursue the philosophy of the limit, in accordance with the ethics of alterity, and try to move beyond parergonal logics in order to engage what is rendered second. If we want to chart a theory of the body, for example, that both highlights its modern technological construction and suggests what that construction omits, we need to engage in a theory of truth that does not require conformity to accepted technological understandings of the body's reality, but instead remains intentionally open to that which *does not* conform. The truth of theoretical writing in such a trajectory has a special character: rather than closing in on the truth, capturing it in some theoretical and signifying framework, it creates an opening for as-yet-inconceivable, unsignified, and perhaps even unsayable truths. This is a form of writing about which Deleuze and Guattari (1987) speak: 'Writing has nothing to do with signifying. It has to do with surveying, mapping, even realms that are yet to come' (4–5). This matter of fostering an alterity that is sensitive to opening spaces for ethical encounters with that which is other is crucial to appreciating the body's potential for transcending the discourses that otherwise constitute it.

So the truth of a theory in the philosophy of the limit lies not in the accuracy of its fit with accepted, socially constructed experiences of reality, but in its capacity to open a space for alternative encounters with, and productions of, reality. Rather than grounding truth in familiar conceptual frameworks and practices, this is a concept of truth that carries us to the very border of strangeness, to paraphrase Wallace Stegner (as cited in Martin 1999, 41). The theory works by opening its user to that which the user's parergonal logic renders second. Alterity to that which is second allows revelation of the parergonal logic. This is a concept of truth that Heidegger has described as *aletheia*, unconcealment. This unconcealment looks simultaneously backwards and forwards, as it were: backward at the parergonal logic, by virtue of appreciating what it omits, and forward from the parergonal logic, by way of openness to the potential of departure.

In this concept of truth, unconcealed otherness remains free by virtue of the theory's reluctance to define or delineate the precise nature of otherness in a way that nevertheless remains attentive to the other's presence or manner of becoming. In other words, what truth may occur in the enactment of the theories developed here resides not in the precision of the correspondence between the words on the page and some external reality, but in the event of unconcealment in the reader or in other deconstructive, contemplative practices that this text may facilitate. Here the truth is decidedly outside my text and my theory. For this reason, the theory of the body in chapter 2 should be understood not as a complete theory of the body, but as a partial and tentative tool for becoming attuned to what the body is and might become.

Deleuze and Guattari (1983) are blunt: 'Artaud puts it well: all writing is so much pig shit – that is to say, any literature that takes itself as an end or sets ends for itself, instead of being a process that "ploughs the crap of being and its language," transports the weak, the aphasiacs, the illiterate ... The only literature is that which places an explosive device in its package, fabricating a counterfeit currency, causing the superego and its form of expression to explode' (134).

Intertextuality

I invoke many diverse writers in this book. My combination of these various authors is both pragmatic and meant to reflect the reality that this book seeks to elicit. I am attempting here to create an analytical tool that can recall what the modern technological way of being has sacrificed. This calls for an eclectic dynamic that extracts useful concepts from the authors, rather than deferring to the authority of their *oeuvres*. Their works cannot be brought together in a unified gestalt. They have their differences. Nevertheless, we can draw threads selectively from each and reweave them together in ways that are appropriate to this study. My loyalty is not to the objective history of concepts and their 'creators,' but to operationalizing *some* of their inspirations. I doubt that any of the authors would mind, too much. Deleuze and Guattari actually invite such an approach. As Brian Massumi, in his *User's Guide to Capitalism and Schizophrenia: Deviations from Deleuze and Guattari*, points out: 'Most of all, the reader is invited to lift a dynamism *out* of the book and incarnate it in a foreign medium, whether painting or politics [I am adding physical education]. Deleuze and Guattari delight in stealing from other disciplines, and they are more than happy to return the favour. Deleuze's own image for a concept [is] not as a brick but as a "tool box." He calls his kind of philosophy "pragmatics" because its goal is the invention of concepts that do not add up to a system of belief or an architecture of propositions that you either enter or you don't, but instead pack a potential in the way a crowbar in a willing hand evokes an energy of prying' (1992, 8). As Deleuze and Guattari (1983) say: 'Reading a text is never a scholarly enterprise in search of what is signified, still less a highly textual exercise in search of a signifier. Rather it is a productive use of the literary machine, a montage of desiring-machines, a schizoid exercise that extracts from the text its revolutionary force' (106).

So I draw selectively on the works of a variety of writers not to develop a unified and comprehensive system of thought that remains in some way true to traditional interpretations of their work, but rather to pry open the technology of physical fitness in order to consider critically what it tries to produce. In so doing, I want to make a clearing that might foster the deep, indeed revolutionary, freedom that remains concealed in the modern technology of physical fitness. The theory of the body developed in chapter 2 has that very practical goal. My commitment to alterity is a commitment to deconstructing practices that limit the appearance of things, especially the body, in order that there may be a compassionate openness (Glass 1995) to the profound potential for freedom (Nancy 1993). I use the works of these thinkers to aid such opening. Compassionate opening is more important to me than fidelity to the canons of the masters. My use of their texts, therefore, is highly selective.

That selective approach is perhaps most important in my use of Heidegger, who has been criticized most appropriately for his troubling relationship with Nazism and, more contentiously, for the reader's suspicion that every word that he wrote and every idea to which he alludes leads to fascism. The ideas that I cite are taken on their own, removed from the whole of Heidegger's philosophy and life, implemented here as tools for freedom. I *appropriate* the words of Heidegger and others only insofar as they aid my critical project. If the reader takes this project, which I propose as an experiment in what Foucault (1983a) has called non-fascist living (xiii), as a fascist program simply because Heidegger's other ideas, ideas not written here, were fascist, then it is the reader who insinuates fascism in this text by appealing to his or her version of Heidegger and imposing it on this text. In other words, I offer at face value the specific uses that I make of Heidegger and others as I present them here, without reference to the authority of the writers, to their work in general, and to the edifices of scholarship that surround them.

In this way my use of these authors is more like collage than cumulative exegesis. This gathering of texts is, as Deleuze and Guattari say, a matter of 'making use of everything that came within range,' 'an intensive way of reading, in contact with what is outside [each] book [or author], as a flow, meeting other flows' (Stivale 1998, as cited 78). While the life-works of these thinkers are often significantly at odds with each other, elements of them do have what Goethe has called 'elective affinities,' which Guattari said can be drawn on to 'forge new analytical instruments, new concepts; because it's not the shared traits that count there, but rather the transversality, the crossing of [possibilities] that constitute a subjectivity that [can be] incarnated' (Stivale 1998, 196). As Massumi (1992) points out: 'The question is not, Is it true? But, Does it work? What new thoughts does it make possible to think? What new emotions does it make possible to feel? What new sensations and perceptions does it open in the body?' (8).

I select elements of the work of various writers as tools for this project. No writing exists in isolation – all writing is intertextual and draws on the works of many others. Indeed it is meaningless without them. I intend the extensive quotations in this book to draw attention to the ways in which the analysis that I offer here is part of a wide, proliferating, intermingling intertextual activity (Deleuze and Guattari 1983; 1987). My practice of quotation is not a review of literature – a form that pretends to represent comprehensively a field of study against which a book attempts to stand out. Instead I quote in order to make multiple connections with a wider **body** of writing or flow of texts and to de-emphasize the individuality or particularity of this text. I mean this practice to embody in writing what the text argues is true about the body in general. In chapter 2 I develop a theory of the body in the intersections of postmodernism and Zen Buddhism that emphasizes the ways in which bodies are profoundly interconnected and reflective of each other. Writing is an expression of that interconnectedness. I hope that my practice of quotation reflects that dictum.

Outline of This Book

Because scientific conceptions of the body have come to dominate modern understandings of the body in general, and the cultures of physical fitness and physical education in particular, I begin chapter 1 with a discussion of some influential postmodern scholarship in the philosophy of science and technology. Science is commonly understood to be an objective, value-free, and non-political enterprise. In chapter 1 I show how it is actually a value-laden and highly political form of knowledge production that profoundly affects how life unfolds. Technology is frequently presented as an advanced method of making things happen. Drawing particularly on the work of Heidegger, I argue that is itself an aggressive project of resource development that, in conjunction with the power-knowledge of science, transforms life. Similar to ecologists' observations on the disastrous effects that advanced technological exploitation of resources has had on the environment and on other species, I maintain that the application of modern scientific technology to the body can be profoundly harmful.

Chapter 2 proposes a theory of the body that attempts to show how the energy of the body becomes available to socio-cultural manipulations, particularly those of science and technology. In this theory of the body I also try to identify the ways in which the very power of the body that is available for exploitation also harbours the potential to transcend that exploitation. Drawing on the work of Heidegger, Foucault, and Deleuze and Guattari, chapter 2 develops a theory of the body that considers the way in which the structure of movement makes the body accessible to the power of modern science and technology. Invoking the question of alterity from the philosophy of the limit, it suggests how bodily powers both transcend and are subordinated by the power of modern science and technology. Following the work of Robert Glass, I make connections between postmodern and Zen Buddhist theories of transcendence. Chapter 2 closes with thoughts on the ways in which a modern technological approach to the body articulates a will to domination that is ultimately fascist, in Deleuze and Foucault's sense.

Chapter 3 applies the theoretical frameworks of the previous two chapters to the technology of physical fitness, describing the ways in which modernity turns the body into a problem in need of technological solutions. As a textual analysis of the techno-science of physical fitness, it examines five fields of texts that play off each other intertextually:

- government policies and publications on health and fitness
- the texts of academic exercise science
- popular texts of physical fitness
- physical fitness products
- popular representations of the fit body

Chapter 4 analyses how this ensemble describes, inscribes, and prescribes a way of life centred on humanism, egoism, youthism, and phallicism. The analysis calls on Taylor's deconstruction of the cosmology of modernity, defined by the death of God and the ascent of Man: the dominating will of God becomes the dominating will of Man. Domination, I argue, is at the core of the modern project. Mod-

ern cosmology centres on a desire for human and individual sovereignty. While this sovereign quest makes sense out of the technological approach to life, it is an impossible pursuit, a desire for solidity
where there is none. As Buddhist philosophy observes, old age, decay,
and death are inevitable; life is essentially impermanent, and the inability to accept that causes great suffering. The discourse of the physically fit body, especially as it ages, marks a modernist resistance to the
inevitable movement of life. Faced with the inevitable failure of the
modern quest for sovereignty, the technology of physical fitness promises salvation. Here is a soteriology – a theory of salvation – that is
geared to the aggressive management, exploitation, accumulation, and
consumption of individual biological resources rather than a contemplative acceptance of the essential movement of being. Grasping for
permanence, rather than moving with the flow of life, the technology
of physical fitness is ultimately a nihilistic way of passing through life.

The Postscript comments on the spiritual destiny that the technological approach to being and the body suggests. It argues that the
more closely life is made to conform to the scripts of the sovereignty-
seeking technological enterprise, the more it is subjected to the rationality of accumulation and consumption, the closer it comes to a life
of complete subordination, to the total control of phallic desire, and
the more it embodies the nihilism that Heidegger feared was our destiny. Following Foucault's understanding of the productivity of discourse, I propose that this nihilism produces an embodied political
system: body fascism. But nihilism is not a *fait accompli*. The philosophy of the limit suggests that every system, including body fascism,
entails a beyond. Drawing on potentials articulated theoretically in
chapter 2, the Postscript ponders the nature of alterity under body
fascism.

PART ONE:
THEORY

1

Theory of Science:
Practice, Power, Consensus

Science is story-telling.
John Polanyi 2000

Natural Science?

The naturalistic understanding of the technology of physical fitness sees it as a scientifically informed approach to developing the body's capacities. Some technologies, in this view, are more scientifically sound than others. The 'best' are those that are most fully informed by 'good science' – science conducted independent of any political or economic interference. For instance, scientific research on training methods conducted by manufacturers of fitness equipment or by drug companies that could make money from the products whose effectiveness is being researched might be seen as tainted, unless it is conducted under the auspices of properly credentiallized scientists, working at arm's length from the manufacturers of the fitness products and the drugs and publishing the results of their research in properly accredited, independent journals of peer review. In the naturalistic view, the best technology is that which is the most scientifically grounded – free of interference, free of the machinations of power, be they economic, political, or any other kinds of power. In this chapter, I question the independence of science from systems of power in the technology of physical fitness.

What is the relationship between scientific knowledge and power? In his book, *Knowledge and Power: Towards a Political Philosophy of Science*, Joseph Rouse (1987) suggests that they can be understood as essentially separate. (This is the received view, which I call 'naturalis-tic,' in which good science is essentially innocent of political impera-tives) or unified (his political philosophy of science, which conceptual-izes science as essentially political). He says that the received view usually understands three kinds of interaction (13). In the first, knowl-edge is applied in order to gain power: knowledge gives people the ability to control or manipulate phenomena; ignorance leaves them with less control. A second kind of interaction occurs where power thwarts the acquisition of (true) knowledge. In this case, false beliefs get in the way of a true understanding. Critical theorists attack this kind of interaction of power and science for its unexposed ideology; scientific knowledge thus needs to be critiqued and cleansed of its ideological underpinnings. (Horkheimer and Adorno 1972, xii, 3–9). In the third interaction, knowledge has the capacity to 'liberate us from the repressive effects of power. It can uncover the distortions power imposes and unmask the disguises that permit power to operate with reduced interference' (Rouse 1987, 13). An example is physiological research that avoids sexist bias and looks at the 'objective truth' of the human body in an attempt to afford women freedom from their tradi-tional physical oppression – see, for example, Ken Dyer 1982 and Shangold 1988.

Rouse points out that power and knowledge remain discrete in the received views, which conceive the epistemological status of knowl-edge claims as independent of the operations of power – the best way to pursue knowledge is to remove power from its production. That is, power can influence what we believe, but considerations of power are entirely irrelevant to which of our beliefs are true, which of these we know to be true, and what justifies their status as knowledge. The work-ing assumption is that inquiry freed from political pressure is the best route to knowledge but that ultimately an epistemological assessment of that achievement must not refer to the intervention of power either in support of or in opposition to knowledge. Similarly, power may or may not serve knowledge or draw on it; it remains power all the same. In their constitution as power and as knowledge, power and knowledge are (in principle) free from one another's influence (13).

Take, for example, the received view on scientific knowledge about women's participation in sport and other demanding recreational physi-cal activities. It claims that knowing the truth of women's bodies is devoid of any gender politics, of the play of power between feminists and patriarchs; feminist concerns may have brought the issue to the fore, but the epistemological status of contemporary non-sexist knowledge of women's bodies is independent of any political program. Truth, it is thought, lies outside these politics. Likewise, patriarchal or feminist power may employ scientific knowledge, but neither in any way depends on such knowledge; that is, neither derives its political logic from scientific knowledge. For instance, while feminist scholars of sport call on existing physiological science to give credence to their claim that women are physically capable of participation in sport, their political program is not the product of their physiological studies. Indeed, feminist philosophies of science are largely the product of feminist analysis and activism from other domains as they have been brought to bear on science. In other words, feminist politics are not the product of scientific knowledge. And as for a philosophy of knowledge in the received view of science, the truth of a statement is independent of the political forces that might have guided its generation. As Rouse says: 'The truth may set us free or it may not, but it remains truth all the same. The point in each case is the same: power can influence our motivation to achieve knowledge and can deflect us from such achievement, but it can play no constructive role in determining what knowledge is' (14). The received view also sees power as repressive, a negative force that prohibits, censors, constrains, and coerces (16). Hubert Dreyfus and Paul Rabinow (1983) have described this understanding as 'a tradition which sees power only as constraint, negativity and coercion. As a systematic refusal to accept reality, as a repressive instrument, as a ban on truth, the forces of power prevent or at least distort the formation of knowledge. Power does this by suppressing desire, fostering false consciousness, promoting ignorance, and using a host of other dodges. Since it fears the truth, power must repress it' (129).

Foucault (1980a) has argued against this 'repressive hypothesis' (10), saying that power is actually productive, creative of desire, consciousness, and knowledge. Indeed it is the capacity to produce reality along certain lines that makes modern power so potent. In this way power is positive, though not always productive of ethico-political realities that we might consider 'positive.'

Rouse (1987) sketches as well an alternative account of power and knowledge, arguing that the received view 'leads us to overlook important ways power is exercised today and to misunderstand both scientific practices and their political effects' (17). This alternative account portrays science, first, as embedded in a matrix of power relations, as part of historical ways of relating to the world. Science engages in social and cultural processes, grounded in society's sense of what counts as important knowledge and valued for its contribution to the organization of society and life in general; thus scientific knowledge is politically grounded.[1] Second, science is technologically based – engaged in shaping, indeed changing the world. Modern science is not just a passive, contemplative description of the world; it produces knowledge by acting on the world. Experimental science does not simply observe the world in its 'natural' state; it manipulates the world in order to know it. 'Scientists produce phenomena: many of the things they study are not "natural" events but are very much the result of artifice' (Rouse 1987, 23). Experimental science takes place in a *laboratory*, Rousse notes, not an *observatory*. For example, practitioners produce scientific knowledge about the cardiovascular training effect has been produced by manipulating humans and animals. They measure cardiovascular systems of untrained subjects (usually either rats or people); they compel subjects to exercise at specific intensities over specific amounts of time and then measure them again. They take the difference in values as indicators of a training effect.

Knowledge of the training effect can emerge only with substantial interference in the lives of the rats and the people being studied. And this knowledge depends on a host of technologies: both exercise technological equipment (for example, treadmills, cycling or rowing ergometers) and measuring technologies (such as the Beckman metabolic cart). Thus scientific knowledge is not antecedent to technological interventions but is actually the product of such interventions. It is the product of the power of technology to generate phenomena. Similarly, technology is the product of scientific study, itself the result of previous technological innovations, which emerge from scientific study – and so on.

Science is intimately related to the politics of the culture, which determines what constitutes knowledge and which affects the technological production of the realities that science makes. Thus power is not a force external to the truths of science but is at the very heart of a scientific way of relating to, of producing, reality. This productive philosophy of science contradicts the popular view that scientific knowledge is simply an apolitical representation; in this philosophy, science renders an account of the world that it has been responsible for making.

This chapter looks, first, at science as a practice that *produces* reality; second, at the power of scientific texts; and third, at how science, through its texts, regulates consensus.

Science as Practice

This section summarizes the philosophical arguments behind Rouse's alternative account of science, specifically as he calls on Kuhn, Heidegger, and Foucault. I use testing of physical fitness to illustrate this account. I refer specifically to the Canadian Physical Activity, Fitness and Lifestyle Appraisal (CPAFLA), a widely used and scientifically credible technology for testing fitness; its development and administration are overseen by the Canadian Society for Exercise Physiology (CSEP), which is the hegemonic academic body for exercise science in Canada, funded by the government of Canada.[2]

Understanding science as productive of reality rather than as merely descriptive of it is understanding science as practice (Rouse 1987, 26–40). The pre-eminent philosopher of science as practice has been Thomas Kuhn, notably in his book *The Structure of Scientific Revolutions* (1970). Rouse says that Kuhn has often been misunderstood. Many readers have seen him as a philosopher of science preoccupied with theoretical paradigms and the ways in which scientific knowledge is thoroughly grounded in the hegemonic processes of theoretical establishments: scientific research takes place under established theoretical paradigms, which occasionally undergo revolutionary changes. Kuhn himself has argued against this centrality of *theoretical* paradigms and said that science is produced more by *practical* paradigms – habitual, practical, paradigmatic ways of dealing with the world. The theoretical emphasis suggests that scientists share, usually uncritically, a set of beliefs about the nature of what they are studying and how they should study it; there is a theoretical consensus. 'Normal science' occurs within this consensus; 'revolutionary science,' in contrast, engages in new theoretical paradigms and pursues research in accordance with the new theory. Gradually more and more scientists come to share the same theoretical beliefs, a consensus emerges, and revolutionary becomes normal science.

A more radical view has it that science works within practical paradigms – habitual, standardized ways of dealing with the world, conducting research, publishing, and so on. What is agreed on is not a set of theoretical beliefs, but rather modes of practical engagement, accepted ways of solving problems and finding solutions. Scientific knowledge is the product of scientists' familiarity with techniques and accepted ways of manipulating phenomena. This is the practicality of scientific knowledge – 'normal science' takes place within accepted practices, which are the product of tacit and relatively unreflective agreement. Rouse (1987) writes: 'Philosophical readers of Kuhn have usually equated scientific revolutions with major conceptual and theoretical changes in a field. We can see, however, that this association need not be the case for Kuhn. New instruments, techniques, or phenomena can cause equally fundamental changes in the way research is done within a given field. A good example is the development of recombinant DNA techniques in biology. These techniques dramatically changed the questions one could ask, and the kinds of answers one could expect within some areas of molecular genetics' (38).

Similarly, in exercise physiology, the technology of metabolic measuring devices such as the Beckman metabolic cart sets the parameters for asking questions and expectations about answers about the body's response to exercise. The technology itself develops a path of research. The practicalities of measuring metabolic exchanges and the widespread acceptance of that practice in exercise physiology circles constitute a practical paradigm for understanding the physiology of exercise. Questions and answers are tied to such technology. The fact that technologies change over time does not alter the dependence of scientific research on technology.

Particular technologies determine in advance what can be known. For instance, the CPAFLA is part of a practical paradigm for studying physical fitness; specifically, it surfaced within an epidemiological context that has been subsequently applied to an individual context. The government of Canada sponsored the National Conference on Fitness and Health in 1972; the gathering called for a comprehensive scientific assessment of the physical fitness of Canadians and produced twenty-four recommendations (Canada 1972). The Canadian Public Health Association originally developed the fitness test and fully implemented it in the Canadian Fitness Survey (1981), initiated and funded by Fitness and Amateur Sport Canada. A technology designed to produce epidemiological knowledge – knowledge geared to the medico-scientific management of disease in populations – is applied to the production of knowledge about individuals. The test is used for individuals because it is there: it employs an established technique, and scientists are practically accustomed to it. The CPAFLA, which is similar to the methods of fitness testing recommended by the American College of Sports Medicine (1993), is a paradigmatic practice among Canadian exercise scientists interested in promoting physical fitness in the general population.[3]

The practical paradigms of science are not only technical – in the sense of the technicalities of recombinant DNA or data collection in the CPAFLA – they are also based in the practicalities of modes of human engagement in the world. Scientific paradigms come from engaged ways of being-in-the-world – the ways in which we deal with the future. For instance, scientific research on AIDS is carried out within human contexts that include citizens' concern for the sick, capitalist drug companies' desire to make money, and individual scientist's search for fame.

More generally, from the work of Heidegger, Rouse argues that part of the formal structure of the engagement of human beings in the world is futurality. In *Being and Time*, Heidegger (1927) argues that an essential element in the human mode of being (*Dasein*) is 'historicality' – temporality, as constituted in the trinity of future, past, and present. And a crucial part of futurality is finding meaning in life in terms of possibilities for the future as they emerge in the present out of the past (434–9). Heidegger says that it is only through engagement with the future that people grasp reality and sense how to act (193). Understanding the future is not just one option among a variety of understandings – for example, understanding the past, present, *or* future. Practical engagement with future possibilities is the formal ground of any understanding whatsoever, including the scientific. Rouse explains this point of Heidegger's: '[Humans] understanding themselves in terms of possibilities is ... a condition of the possibility of there being an understanding of being (i.e. any disclosure of beings) at all. The possibilities in terms of which Dasein understands itself are not something distinct from its understanding of the world, including "nature." To understand oneself in terms of possibilities is to understand the world as a field of possible action. This is the configuration within which anything becomes intelligible, not just Dasein ... Meaning is a "formal" condition on the intelligibility of beings rather than a substantive characteristic of some particular being' (183).

Rouse applies this point to the engagement of science, saying that it too is engaged in this fundamental human temporal structure: caring about the future in terms of possibilities. Science makes possible caring in such a way that *particular* future possibilities emerge. The practical paradigms of science therefore involve the ways in which it engages future possibilities. Indeed it is that engagement with the future that makes science meaningful or worthwhile. The future control of disease, for instance, is essential to the engagement of preventive medicine: scientific research in preventive medicine is geared to this practical concern about controlling disease in the future. We can see this link between scientific knowledge and concern for future health, for example, in a letter (15 March 1995) sent to graduates of the University of Toronto signed by a professor from the Department of Preventive Medicine and the director of Alumni Development in which they encourage the recipients to participate in a large-scale pan-Canadian study 'The Canadian Study of Diet, Lifestyle and Health': 'Every year thousands of Canadians develop diseases such as cancer, heart disease, and diabetes. These conditions appear to be related to the way we live, to our eating and drinking habits, and to our exercise patterns. Therefore, it is thought that by modifying our diet and lifestyle it might be possible both to prevent some of these diseases and to allow us to live more of our lives in good health. Researchers at several Canadian universities (Alberta, British Columbia, Toronto, Western Ontario) are proposing to carry out jointly one of the largest studies to date to investigate the effects of eating patterns and other lifestyle factors on *future* health' (emphasis added). This letter reflects a major aspect of modern science – namely, that it is not simply a disengaged reflection on nature, but is conducted out of concern with the ways in which it can engage nature in order to produce life along certain lines (in this case, purportedly, with diminished incidence of disease). The program of research mentioned here is meaningful only insofar as it has a possible effect on the future; if it had no such bearing, it would not take place.

Certainly, the entire field of health promotion is futural. For instance, the World Health Organization defines the field as a process that increases individuals and communities' control over their future health.[4] Government interest in health promotion derives from an economic concern for the future – that spiralling medical costs will render 'health care' untenable – and sees health promotion as a way of dealing with health care in less expensive ways. Scientific research in 'lifestyle management' – one of the 'four action areas' of health promotion (Kickbusch 1994, 12) – is concerned entirely with the relationship between present behaviour, future health, and possibilities for behavioural change. Consequently, the CPAFLA assesses present levels of fitness and risks to future health and prescribes ways of living an active life. The second recommendation of the National Conference on Fitness and Health in 1972 was to change Canadian values and ways of life (Canada 1972, 126).

My point is that the science of physical fitness, exemplified by the CPAFLA, is similar to other forms of scientific knowledge in its concern for the future and for the transformation of human life such that the future may unfold along certain lines. It is not a detached, politically neutral way of producing knowledge about individual bodies and ways of life; it exists as a method of engaging and changing lives, to align them with both official political and economic policies of government (as in health promotion) and less explicit, but nevertheless powerful, politics of the body. Hence scientific knowledge 'must be understood in terms of its use' (Rouse 1987, 126). Medico-scientific knowledge that is not useful is, well, useless.

This concern for the future and for the creation of scientific knowledge that is useful for making possibilities unfold in certain ways governs future possibilities. This is a realm of government described by Foucault: '"Government" did not refer only to political structures or to the management of states ... the legitimately constituted forms of political or economic subjection, but also modes of action, more or less considered and calculated, which were destined to act upon the possibilities of action of other people. *To govern, in this sense, is to structure the possible field of action of others'* (Foucault 1983b, 221, as quoted in Rouse 1987, 185).[5] Science governs in this sense, structuring individuals' possible field of action. Rouse observes: 'A field of action is constituted both by material surroundings and technical capabilities and by a shared understanding of what it makes sense to do and to be in those surroundings. Scientific practice is political in the sense that it helps structure our field of possible action in both ways' (185). This is not political in the same way that legislation and courts of law are political. It is political in the sense that it sets parameters for what is meet and right, given what science has rendered possible. More and more legislation is created on the basis of what science has laid out in the realm of the possible. In many countries, there is legislation that deals, for example, with genetic engineering, use of human tissue, and regulation of telecommunications. Rouse points out that the scientific revolution brought about much more than intellectual changes: 'This revolution changed what was at issue in being human. The Cartesian subject of modern philosophy emerged from reflection on how such a physical order could be comprehended and known; the relation between human beings and the divine took on new shapes; the problem emerged of whether and how physical and moral descriptions of persons were compatible; and both the gendering of nature and the sexual imagery of our knowledge of it were revised. These were not only intellectual changes. They were connected to transformations in political relations and institutions, the creation of new religious practices, and the emergence of new forms of economic behaviour and social interaction' (186).

Science is political in how it affects the way in which people relate to nature and to each other. That is the productive power of science. And its 'real-life' productive power lies in the way in which it moves out of the laboratory and into daily life. The CPAFLA, administered in universities, fitness clubs, recreation centres and employee fitness programs, is one instance of the insinuation of the power of science into everyday life.

I invoked above Rouse's argument that science does not simply observe nature and comment on it. Science actually provokes nature to appear in certain ways; as we see in the difference between the *observatory* and the *labora*tory. Its capacity to provoke nature is fundamental to its power: 'The development of scientific knowledge is rooted in the construction and manipulation of phenomena through which we develop new skills and uncover new truths and possibilities for truth' (Rouse 1987, 211). But the broadly *political* power of science lies in the way in which the power that goes to work in the laboratory subsequently extends outside it: '[Scientific] developments become disseminated into the world outside the laboratory by standardizing scientific techniques and equipment and by adjusting nonscientific practices and situations to make them amenable to the employment of scientific materials and practices. The result is that the world is increasingly a made world, in the sense that it reflects the systematic extension of ... technical capacities, the equipment they employ, and the phenomena they make manifest' (211).

Chapter 3 below looks at how power extends out of the exercise laboratory to the wider world in the technology of physical fitness. Because it is through texts that scientific knowledge is negotiated between scientists as well as among practitioners and the public, we need to look at the relationship between scientific *texts* and the reality that they describe. We also must consider the theory of the body that those texts both assume and endeavour to reproduce in the lives of the people who use the technology of physical fitness. So, in the next section, I develop a theory of scientific texts using examples from the exercise sciences. Chapter 2 proposes a theory of the body that chapter

3 and 4 apply to deconstruct the operation of power in the technology of physical fitness.

Power in Scientific Texts

The 'usual,' natural reading of scientific texts is naïve. It takes texts as transparent, objective representations of natural reality. It finds the value of the text in its truthfulness, the degree to which it accurately represents reality. But such a valuation does not take into account the wider socio-cultural value of texts and their ethico-political implications. The philosophy of the limit that I outlined above in the Introduction seeks to see through the ostensibly purely descriptive claim of texts and understand them as distinctly political systems that circumscribe, or more accurately, in the case of the scientific texts of the technology of physical fitness, *prescribe* the limits of the real through particular logics of parergonality.

I derive the map for my analysis of the philosophy of the limit in scientific texts from work in the philosophy, sociology, and anthropology of science, specifically the work of Latour (1987), Bazerman (1988), and Shapin and Schaffer (1985). Focusing on Latour and Bazerman, I argue that scientific texts constitute a socio-cultural system. By appealing to Gramsci's theory of hegemony (Shapin and Schaffer 1985; Williams 1977; 1980) and to Bourdieu's theories of cultural reproduction and symbolic power (Bourdieu 1979, 1990), I propose that this socio-cultural system hegemonically produces reality. Through a fairly standard program of rhetoric and symbolic violence, scientific texts hegemonize particular philosophies of Nature and, in the technology of physical fitness, the body.

A standard textbook on exercise physiology includes the following words and graph for understanding the training effect of physical exercise:

A schema is proposed to summarize adaptive changes in active muscle that accompany a change in VO_2max with endurance training. As shown in figure 21.6. aerobic capacity increases about 15 to 30% over the first 3 months of intensive training and may rise by as much as 50% over a 2-year period. When training stops, the aerobic capacity decreases toward the pre-training level. The effect is even more impressive for the aerobic enzymes of the Krebs cycle and the electron transport chain. These enzymes, which facilitate carbohydrate and lipid breakdown, increase rapidly and substantially throughout the training period in both fibre types and subdivisions. Conversely a large portion of this metabolic adaptation is lost within a few weeks after training ceases. The number of muscle capillaries increases throughout training. This adaptation to blood supply is probably lost at a relatively slow rate when training stops. (McArdle, Katch, and Katch 1996, 401)

This passage appears in the textbook as a simple explanation of how exercise physiologists calculate the physical intensity of exercise. It is but one among several hundred similar practical physiological explanations in an 850-page textbook. The volume is geared to physical education students and could serve as a typical reference text for would-be appraisers of physical fitness, higher-level personal trainers, aerobic instructors, and so on.[6] Students typically have to read, understand, and reproduce this physiological knowledge in an examination. The information is relatively simple and straightforward. Instructors expect students to read this text as a transparent, objective, non-political representation of the natural reality of the exercising human body. Having done so, they will have learned what exercise physiology wishes to teach – here, specific effects of endurance training over time.

Ostensibly, readers take this information and use it to organize the exercise behaviour of their future clients or students. This information will therefore affect people, and so the text is socio-culturally significant. Because it (in)forms human practice – it exists in order to do so; it is not a purely speculative text – it is not simply a socially detached account of a physiological study, but an active part of the process of organizing human life. Physical educators who have learned about the effects of endurance training will encourage people to bring their bodies to such a threshold on a regular basis – a task that can be quite demanding physically, psychically, and socially. Moreover, they will encourage clients to think of themselves, their bodies, in terms of the long-term effects of endurance training and of the negative implications of discontinuing it. The text therefore informs a significant intrusion into the practices and meanings of human lives. Obviously, there should be political and ethical concern wherever life is subjected to such intrusion.

The social nature of scientific texts has been a major topic in the history, philosophy, and sociology of science for the last twenty-five years or so (Pickering 1992; 1995). One school sees scientific texts as realist representations of nature. While their production has a social dimension (the sociology of the laboratory, the scientific publishing industry, and so on), a correct correspondence between the inscriptions of the texts (words, numbers, scientific symbols, charts, graphs, and so on) and the objects that the inscriptions are meant to represent is still possible and, indeed is often the case. In other words, the 'truthfulness' of the text – the validity of the representation of the reality that it describes – is independent of the social organization of science and its representational practices. Anti-realists argue, in contrast, that science is social to its core – scientific knowledge is essentially a textual play of socially constructed signifiers, more or less (depending on how radical the theory is) independent of nature, if there is any such thing as nature without signifiers.

The position that I propose here does not attempt to resolve the realist–anti-realist debate. It allows that various scientific knowledges *may* accurately represent nature: I do not contest, for example, the verity of the concept of the endurance training effect. Science has been immensely successful at controlling nature; science 'works.' In the exercise sciences, for instance, scientific knowledge about oxygen transport and elimination of blood lactates has led to training techniques that have improved use of the body for swimming faster. Likewise biomechanical knowledge of the human gait when running may have led to better running shoes, thereby decreasing injuries and making running more comfortable. And standardized tests of physical fitness allow people to judge their level of fitness and to strive for improvements on that basis. Scientific methods for determining levels of exercise intensity have made it possible for people to optimize their exercise programs and to accomplish basic physical fitness or competitive athletic goals. Clearly, the representations of exercise science have been effective in getting the human body to submit to the human will. There must therefore be some connection between such representations and the 'natural' reality of the human body.

My argument here is that while science is very effective at making nature conform to human desires, it is but one way of understanding it. All but the most dogmatic of scientists would agree that there are many ways of seeing, representing, and understanding nature. There have been various aesthetics of nature throughout the history of fine art. Nature has been rendered in poetry. And there is the breathtaking view of Nature that one sees while canoeing northern lakes or hiking in the mountains. Likewise, nature's human body has been seen in art, rendered in poetry, and experienced in human movements such as running, climbing, and sex. But science represents nature quite differently from the representations and experiences of art, poetry, and movement. The question that I address here concerns the nature of scientific textual representation and the way in which it influences the 'reading' of nature.

I am concerned here about the *texts* of science. For it is with texts, and not with scientific experiments, that the vast majority of people (both scientist and lay) interact. Texts (in)form human practice; it is exposure to the text, not to the host of scientific procedures that lie behind it, that lead exercise consultants to recommend endurance training. People develop scientific understanding through texts; while many of us have various levels of scientific understanding of the world and of our bodies, few of us ever actually engage in the experimental work that is said to produce scientific understanding. And Latour (Latour and Woolgar 1986) points out that even experimental researchers base most of their understanding not on the experiments that they have themselves observed, but on previous work written up by others. Because experimental science is a cumulative enterprise, with each experiment based on the written results of previous experiments in related fields, including research on the operation, capacity, and validity of the laboratory instruments used in experiments, *no* scientist actually observes the entire experimental process. All scientists depend on what Kristeva (1980) calls the intertextuality of texts, thus creating their scientific texts out of other texts.[7]

Science is preoccupied with the production of written texts. Indeed, without its texts, there is no science. Shapin and Schaffer point out that the epistemological basis of an experimental fact lies in its public nature: a scientific fact is what is accepted by a scientific community. Historically, the scientific community gathered round, watched the experiment, and came to some agreement as to what happened in it. Nowadays, of course, this is impossible. Scientific texts substitute for the actual presence of the community at the experimental site (Shapin and Schaffer 1985, 22 ff; Shapin 1994). Because community (peer) agreement lies at the very heart of scientific factuality, and the community can really come together only textually, the text is central to the production, to the existence, of scientific truth.

So there are three good reasons to focus on scientific texts:

- Scientific texts (in)form human practice.
- Each scientific text rests on the backs of myriad other texts.
- Scientific texts constitute the public forum that makes possible the community agreement necessary for the attainment of scientific truth.

But why all this fuss? Do not texts simply represent the experimental events that occurred outside them?

While scientific texts do describe an amalgam of experimental events and other texts, they also reproduce a hegemonic culture of nature, thus narrowing the scope of what humans can think about nature, which the philosophy of the limit calls the logic of parergonality. A complete description of this hegemonic culture of nature is a project beyond the scope of this book – I explore its specific character in regard to the body in chapter 2 and the specific application of that culture in the scientific technology of physical fitness in chapter 3. My concern at this point is not the *content* of the reproduction of hegemonic culture, but the more formal problem of the *way* in which scientific texts reproduce hegemonic culture in their parergonal logic.

The concept of 'hegemony,' as developed by Gramsci, describes the *process* that produces social relations of power. This process, while it has its material bases, works in the creation of reality in the consciousness of people, their sense of what constitutes the real. Williams (1980) explains it as follows: 'In any society, in any particular period, there is a central system of practices, meanings and values which we can properly call dominant and effective ... It thus constitutes a sense of reality for most people in the society, a sense of absolute because experienced reality beyond which it is very difficult for most members of the society to move, in most areas of their lives' (38).

People co-operate in the production of the dominant practices, meanings, and values that constitute hegemonic reality. On the whole, they are not forced by some external power to accept a reality that is somehow foreign to them. Hegemonic power is predicated on some level of consensus about what is real and what is not. Scientific texts engage in the hegemonic production of reality, by developing a culture of consensus.

In this way modern scientific texts are unlike pre-modern texts. The Christian predecessors of scientific texts derived their authority, their sense of natural reality, from what they perceived to exist above, ultimately from God, who revealed himself through holy writ and sacraments. Authority over what constituted reality was thought to be beyond human, external to their views of the subjects of reality. But with the advent of modern science, the concept of authority changed from being external to internal, from God to humans. As Shapin and Schaffer (1985) suggest, this shift from external authority to the more 'democratic' development of consensus constituted the true source of disagreement in seventeenth-century England between the old-fashioned philosopher Thomas Hobbes and the modern experimental scientist Robert Boyle.

Regulating Consensus

The correct take on nature, in modern science, is the product of agreement. Latour (1987), Latour and Woolgar (1986), Shapin and Schaffer (1985), Shapin (1994), and Bazerman (1988) have focused on the social processes that produce these scientific agreements. Where there is little agreement, science loses its authority. To hold on to authority, science must maintain a culture of consensus.

Foucault says that with the dawn of modernity political power ceased to be so much a matter of external force and became more a matter of the diffuse internalization of power, an intricate co-optation of the subjects of power in their own subjugation (Foucault 1979; 1980a; 1983; 1988). I suggest that in a not-dissimilar fashion scientific texts co-opt the scientists and the professionals who come under their sway. The whole project is one of trying to achieve and maintain agreement, to keep a consensus about reality. Readers of scientific texts who join in the process are willing to give their consent, to co-operate with the scientific project, because they believe that they have the democratic power to withhold consent, that they are free to dissent if they do not see reality in the way in which the text presents it. But as I argue now, the actual room for dissent is very small. This system works, as Shapin and Schaffer point out, by controlling dissent, by keeping it within boundaries. With consent thus controlled, a hegemonic reality is maintained. Scientific texts come to dominate our sense of reality by securing consent without actually affording substantive opportunity for dissent.

Latour and Woolgar (1986) say that the actual work of science is a matter of separating facts from artefacts. Because the attainment of agreement is essential to the truth value of a text, texts actively engage in the social process of securing agreement about what is a fact and what is an artefact. Developing scientific consensus is a social process, which is not to say that it is a *purely* social process. Nature does place some constraints on what can possibly emerge as a viable textual representation of it. Ludwig Fleck described these as the 'passive linkages' that natural phenomena place on the scientific task of representation (Bazerman 1988, 312). The social activity of working towards consensus in scientific textual representation is limited by the phenomenon being described. For instance, when exercise physiologists settle on the phenomenon of the anaerobic threshold as an indicator of exercise intensity, the character of oxygen constrains what they say about the threshold. The social process of achieving consensus takes place within the context of such passive natural constraints.

While scientific facts about nature may indeed have some truth value, their textual production emerges in an *agonistic* process. Scientists play textual statements off each other: 'Facts are constructed through operations designed to effect the dropping of modalities which qualify a given statement' (Latour and Woolgar 1986, 237). Textual statements compete with each other. This is a crucial point: scientific facts are the products of competing arguments, of a combat that produces winners and losers. And Bazerman brings a fine point to this. Because very few people actually 'see' the scientific experiment, it is not by viewing the play of nature that the scientific community declares a winner and achieves consensus, but rather by considering the play of texts. Even where there are a number of replicated experiments conducted, the interplay of the rhetorics of the *texts* of the replicated experiments leads to possible consensus, not the *actual witnessing* of experiments.[8]

To achieve consensus, to get the scientific community to agree, scientific texts must be persuasive. And it is in the techniques of persuasion that the hegemonic, culturally reproductive nature of scientific texts shows. Synthesizing the work of Bazerman, Latour and Woolgar, and Shapin and Schaffer, we see three interrelated elements in this social strategy of persuasion:

- use of rhetoric to compel the reader to agree
- textual closure that limits the reader's perception and reasoning
- concealment of the social nature of the text such that it appears as a non-social, transparent representation of nature – in short, innocent of any cultural 'interference'

The first claim of a scientific text is that it is an honest representation of experimental events – the text is not lying. Bazerman (1988) says that one rhetorical strategy is to establish *ethos* – 'that the author/observer is a credible witness, following all proper procedures thoughtfully and carefully' (140). Academic credentials serve this purpose, proving that the author has negotiated the socially prescribed indoctrination into the values of the academy. For instance, the *American College of Sports Medicine's Resource Guidelines for Exercise Testing and Prescription* (American College of Sports Medicine, or ACSM, 1993) credentiallizes itself by listing the names of the editors, along with their academic degrees and university affiliation, and lists the forty-seven reviewers along with their academic degrees. Five of the six editors and twenty-three of the forty-seven reviewers are fellows of the ACSM. Credentials, however, are not sufficient for persuasion. Because in science 'seeing is believing,' the reader does not simply trust the credentiallized author's privileged experience of the experiment, but must see the experiment itself through the text.

More important than credentials, usurping their role, and indeed rendering the author invisible, are rhetorical devices that form the text. These devices are intimately connected to the historical development of scientific journals as *the* forum for the resolution of scientific debates. Before the rise of the journal, Bazerman says, the scientific report was more like news, simply saying what happened in an experiment. But as the journal emerged as the centre of debate, simply reporting was insufficient. Journal articles needed to persuade. In a circle of mutual reinforcement, the growth of the journal led to more debate; the more nature was debated, the more debatable it seemed: the more debatable nature appeared, the more important was the debate; the more important the debate, the more important the journal; and so on. In such an intellectual atmosphere, the settling of controversy becomes crucial. The credibility of scientific reality could be at stake. For if scientific truth is based on consensus about the nature of reality, and if consensus becomes ultimately impossible because there are so many conflicting versions of reality, then science itself will be disreputable. For science to succeed, it needs a rhetorical strategy for the management of controversy.

One such managerial rhetoric is to reassure the reader that a given text is 'authentic,' that it accurately represents what happened in the experimental setting. Shapin and Schaffer (1985) refer to this as 'virtual witnessing.' And one of the ways to do this is to include extensive technical details on the experiment. Having much more information than one needs to understand the results of the experiment provides some verisimilitude, as if one were actually present at the experiment, where one is also bombarded with extra data. Including extensive raw data gives the reader the sense that the text is showing everything that happened; it is holding back nothing. As Latour (1987) points out, the reader does not have to believe the author's conclusion; he or she can 'see' the basis for the conclusion in the raw data. Having been shown 'everything that happened in the experiment,' the reader has the impression that he or she is in a position to give or withhold consent. The reader is free to see the experiment as it actually happened. This freedom to 'see' reassures the reader that he or she has choice. Of course, the text does not record everything that happened in the experiment; it records only those things considered important to a very particular scientific vision of reality. Indeed, it usually omits information that could displace scientific reality. The reader is therefore not free. To take an obvious example, very few experiments that use laboratory animals record in any detail their unhappiness or suffering, nor do they attend to the psychological strategies that the technicians employ in order to erase any sympathy/empathy for the animals' unfortunate plight. That sort of information could displace the primacy of the scientific 'take' on reality.

Latour (1987) says that 'when controversies flare up the literature become technical' (21 ff). That manoeuvre, he says, includes a clever quantitative rhetoric of appealing to authority. The more citations a text contains, the more likely it is to be taken seriously (33). For example: the ACSM's manual on exercise testing and prescription lists 1,259 references for forty-seven articles (the highest number of citations per article is 141; the lowest is 0), which is an average of twenty-seven references per average twelve-page article. Part of this rhetoric is the understanding that the reader is welcome to take the presence of many citations *not* as *mere* appeals to authority, but as invitations to read the works cited and judge for himself or herself the validity of the comments based on them. This becomes an impossible numbers game, for if the reader were to trace all the references given – for example, twenty-seven from one article under review – he or she would find in each reference a similar number of references to more articles in each of those references. The believability of each of those in turn depends on following through on their references, which leads to following through on hundreds more, and so on. This is a daunting task that few, if any readers would undertake. This is a rhetoric of intimidation by geometrically expanding intertextual citation. All but the most industrious reader must accept the truthfulness of the intertextual citations.

This is a particularly powerful threat for the non–scientist-professional reader of textbooks, such as physical education students who become physical fitness appraisers, consultants, and teachers. These people believe the texts because of a careful system of referencing that invites them to look at the references and verify the veracity of the science – i.e., to give or withhold consent. They too receive the false impression that they could dissent if they wanted to. But since even a specialist scientist does not have the time to wade through the hundreds of thousands of references that it would take to give faithful consent to a text, certainly the generalist professional, reading in a multitude of scientific disciplines (physiology, biology, biochemistry, biomechanics, nutrition, exercise physiology, statistics, psychology, and sociology, all at an undergraduate level), has no opportunity to do the work necessary to withhold consent. Moreover, it is quite clear to such students that they lack the knowledge and expertise to question their texts. Nevertheless they give consent because they believe that if they had the time and resources to learn all they would need to know in order to be critical, they could dissent. In this way they co-operate in the reproduction of scientific reality.

Now one could argue that the professional reader of scientific textbooks is not part of the (scientific) community that participates in the process of consensus-building about scientific reality. He or she is not, after all, engaged in a critical intellectual relationship with the texts, but merely consumes the texts' facts and procedures. The culture of and burden for developing consensus lies with 'real' scientists. There are two arguments against this exclusion of professional readers. The major argument deals with the practical aspects of hegemonic reality, and the minor one, with the process of convincing professionals of the truth of scientific texts. I deal with the latter first.

While professional readers of scientific texts do not spend much of their time criticizing the science of the texts, they tend to believe them because they trust that research scientists have done so (and Latour has shown that they too are unable to deal with the 'black boxes' of the texts). But professional readers of scientific texts are also usually indoctrinated into the experimental basis of the scientific texts by the lab sessions that are part of their university or college courses and by reading the descriptions of the experiments that justify the facts in their texts. Most professional programs insist that students have some contact with the laboratory so that they will understand (i.e., believe) the texts that come from laboratories; virtually all scientific professional programs have a substantial laboratory element. Having experienced the 'experimental life' (Shapin and Schaffer 1985), albeit at an elementary level, they believe the 'virtual witnessing' of their texts. And the professionals' belief in scientific texts is central to the reproduction of the hegemony of scientific reality. For it is professionals, such as doctors, nurses, pharmacists, dentists, engineers, and physical educators, who put scientific reality into practice And this brings me to the major argument about the role of professionals in the hegemony of scientific reality.

Gramsci says that hegemony is not just an abstract, conceptual matter of meaning and values. Hegemony also entails practices and experiences that engage in a reciprocal relationship with meaning and values. Williams (1980) explains this: 'What I have in mind is the central, effective and dominant system of meanings and values, which are not merely abstract but which are organized and lived. That is why hegemony is not to be understood at the level of mere opinion or mere manipulation. It is a whole body of practices and expectations; our assignments of energy, our ordinary understanding of the nature of man and of his world. It is a set of meanings and values which as they are experienced as practices appear reciprocally confirming' (38).

If the reality produced in scientific texts were nothing more than abstract ponderings of a socially insignificant group of intellectuals, then it would not matter too much; certainly, it would not be hegemonic. But the reality created in scientific texts has shaped virtually every aspect of modern life. Scientific reality is now crucial to the practices of physical education and is the epistemic basis of physical fitness. Professionals put scientific reality into practice, they translate scientific texts into human practices. Physical fitness experts design exercise programs out of the meanings and values that they find in their textbooks.

As Williams emphasizes, the practices and the meanings and values of hegemonic reality are mutually confirming. We can recognize this in the common assertion that 'science works.' The fact that science works makes it very difficult to disagree with the way in which it has set up reality in the first place. For instance, scientific texts provided us with the concept of the anaerobic threshold. These texts have been translated into human practices such as swimming workouts that use the anaerobic threshold to make swimming times faster. This faster swimming confirms the meaning and value of the anaerobic threshold. The science becomes 'real' in this marriage of practice and textuality. But something valuable has been lost: namely, alternative visions of the reality of swimming and the body. These visions might prefer to construe swimming and the body not as productive, performative, linearly temporal, a resource for the professionalization of sport, but rather to make swimming play, liberation, a non-linear, perhaps spiritual, experience of the body that is worthwhile in and of itself, inaccessible to the reality of modern techno-scientific culture, or some such. Such alternative visions become lost in the tight fit of the meaning and value of scientific texts and professional practices.

Excluding alternative categories, meanings, values, priorities, interests, and so on is part of the process of hegemony. Such exclusion is apparent in scientific texts in the way in which they attempt to control the readers' thoughts. The text vies for authority by invoking closure on what the reader may think. Umberto Eco says that closed texts deny the reader the freedom to offer alternative interpretations (Bazerman 1988, 123). Bazerman (1988) explains how a scientific text invokes closure.

(1) That experimental methods and results must be spelled out explicitly and in detail, both to allow replication and comparison of results and to create a plausible virtual experience for readers; (2) That the discourse must be organized around a central claim or sequential series of claims, and the experimental accounts should be structurally and logically subordinated to those claims to serve as a form of experimental proof; (3) That the coordinated series of claims and articles, incorporated into a coherent system, becomes a mutually supporting network framing a way of working, viewing, and thinking, so that reliance on the network becomes an essential cognitive and argumentative resource. Serious arguments can only be cast within the closed system that realizes the mode of perception, activity, thinking, and interchange. Arguments that step out of the closed system are no longer considered properly scientific. (126)

Scientific texts give only the *impression* of free thought and openness to criticism. This is not the open exchange of ideas, visions, or experiences. It is a closed system that sets rhetorical limits to debate. These rhetorical conventions render inadmissible experience and thinking that do not, cannot, conform to the above three requirements. This closure constitutes the logic of parergonality of scientific texts. The texts demand adherence to what is reasonable within their systems. Mark Taylor (1987) comments: 'Reason constitutes itself both theoretically and practically in and through an act of exclusion that is maintained by prohibitions, which every reasonable person deems inviolable. In this way prohibition functions as the condition of the possibility of reason' (131).

And Shapin and Schaffer (1985) have shown that one of the primary functions of scientific learned societies is to set the parameters of debate. Bazerman (1988) points out that most scientific societies publish journals that are reviewed by peers who have consented to the parameters of what is considered acceptable – peers act as the gatekeepers (136). This gatekeeping, Bazerman says, involves the often-complex politics that editorial boards engage in in order to preserve their own points of view. He also points out that only those who are willing to work within the set parameters of debate may publish, and only those who publish are able to conduct 'legitimate' research. By invoking such closure, scientific texts set the boundaries of legitimate debate. They exclude alternative visions of reality. Major dissent in such closed texts is therefore impossible. But because these closed texts allow debate within their boundaries, they appear to allow freedom for dissent. Anyone who wants to participate in science must consent to work within these boundaries. Indeed, much of higher education is an indoctrination into the canon of various boundaried disciplines; it establishes boundaries, a sense of acceptable and unacceptable ways of thinking within particular fields of research. In chapter 3, I offer the example of the science of physical fitness testing's being based on this kind of controlled debate: only those who were willing to consider the body within the objectifying paradigms of the body that are foundational to exercise science helped create the standardized tests of fitness. Dissent is restricted to within the paradigm. Part of the rhetoric that helps reproduce hegemony therefore involves the exclusion of alternatives by maintenance of textual boundaries. People partake in this reproduction by consenting to work within the boundaries as though they were provided sufficient room for dissent.

The scientific society that produces these closed texts aids and abets this closure by its social practices of exclusion. Part of this process of exclusion works by the practice of publishing texts. Scientific journals serve the interests of scientific communities that have agreed on the boundaries of acceptable visions of reality and the parameters of debate. The authority of the journal depends on how carefully it adheres to the established boundaries of the community that it serves. Only those scientific texts that work within those boundaries therefore are acceptable for publication.[9] Editorial boards consequently work as gatekeepers for inclusion or exclusion from the scientific textual community (Merton and Zuckerman 1973). And it is only by virtue of a scientist's history of publication that he or she is acknowledged by the scientific community as a valid critic of the community's work. Consequently, only those who work within the boundaries are deemed acceptable critics. As I mentioned above, five of the six editors of the ACSM's (1993) *Resource Guidelines* and half of the reviewers of the articles for it are FACSMS. Needless to say, this goes a long way to avoiding major dissent within the community. And finally, the great financial cost of conducting much scientific research prohibits all but the most established (who become established by working within the closed world of scientific textuality) from engaging in research. And Latour (1987) argues that even within the boundaries of a given science, the high cost of research makes dissent difficult and sometimes impossible. As Kuhn (1970) points out, a fully established science is unlikely to consider radical alternative visions of reality (i.e., revolutionary paradigms).

Scientific communities thus regulate themselves by their social organization and the rhetoric of their texts. Their self-regulation sets the limits of what can be thought, literally contextualizing acceptable visions of reality. By this process of self-regulation, they maintain hegemony.

One last rhetorical manoeuvre needs attention, the most masterful device of them all – the rhetoric of scientific rhetoric concealing itself. With this rhetoric, the socio-cultural nature of scientific texts disappears and reappears as a simple, transparent, realist representation of nature. Because it makes scientific texts seem innocent of anything but the truth, it is a very persuasive manoeuvre. I call it the rhetoric of innocence.

Bazerman (1988) says: 'One peculiar aspect of the accomplishment of scientific discourse is that it appears to hide itself' (14). When we read about the aerobic capacity, we are expected to believe that we are examining the natural facts about aerobic capacity, not a socio-cultural rhetorical text. But while nature's aerobic capacity may indeed exist, we are reading texts, not nature. This disappearance of the text as a socio-cultural system is a rhetorical move with political results. To see

the socio-cultural construction of the text would bring it into disre-
pute. For the fundamental principle of modern science is that we know
nature by looking at *it*. Having seen *nature*, not humanity, we can rest
assured in the knowledge that comes from the sight. Scientific debates
about the reality of nature are supposedly resolved by letting nature
show itself. Shapin and Schaffer (1985) explain this way of thinking:
'What men make, men may unmake; but what nature makes no man
may dispute' (23).

Here is a conundrum for science. Science claims the unequivocal
power that comes from nature's showing itself, innocent of human
interference. But as I argued above, since the real epistemological basis of scientific facts is the social hegemonizing practice of securing
consensus, scientific texts must be all too humanly rhetorical. To claim
the revelatory power of innocent nature, science must hide the guilt of
human agency, and it must do so with the guilty hand of the texts
themselves. Just as Heraclitus said that 'Nature loves to hide itself'
(Fragment 125), so too the textuality of science. Science hides its guilt
behind the innocent face of nature. While it does so by nothing more
than a leap of faith (a naïve belief in the transparency of texts), it
serves an essential rhetorical function – to free scientific texts of their
socio-cultural foundations. This rhetoric of innocence allows science
to appear to transcend quietly the hurly-burly of the essentially political nature of all human activity.[10]

Scientists and professionals co-operate in the reproduction of hegemonic reality. Yet they do so without admitting as much, even to
themselves. They claim to be simply in the business of telling the
world what nature has shown them. When politics is allowed to hide
this way, their reproduction is that much more effective. The political
(hegemonic) creation of reality is naturalized in scientific texts and
ensuing professional practices. While techno-science clearly has the
power to manipulate the natural world, its most significant power –
which gives it its power of manipulation, which gets people to co-
operate in the actual production of techno-scientific manipulation (not
only of the natural environment, but also of people and bodies) – is
what Bourdieu calls symbolic power.

Symbolic power, writes Bourdieu, is the power to define reality
(Bourdieu 1979; Bourdieu and Passeron 1990). Because the production
of reality lies at the very heart of hegemony, this power is indispensable to the reproduction of hegemonic culture. The power of science is
the power to create reality first symbolically and then reciprocally in

practice (cf. above, regarding the reciprocity of meaning and practice; this is the mutuality of scientists and professionals, the union of techno- and science). Scientific texts create their symbolic power by delimiting what is acceptable as scientific reality.

In science, symbolic power is actually the power to do 'symbolic violence,' which Bourdieu explains as follows: 'Every power to exert symbolic violence, i.e. every power which manages to impose meanings and to impose them as legitimate by concealing the power relations which are the basis of its force, adds its own specifically symbolic force to these power relations' (Bourdieu and Passeron 1990, 4).

The legitimacy of scientific representation lies in its supposedly transparent, non-political representation of nature. But as the philosophy, sociology, and anthropology of science I have been citing suggest, scientific texts are not simply representations of nature but *also* social and political texts. And as I have been arguing, the legitimacy of science is achieved precisely 'by concealing the power relations which are its source.' The power of scientific texts is the power to do violence, by creating a limited sense of reality, by co-opting people into believing in this reality, and by hiding the fact that it is doing so. It is this hiddenness that makes scientific texts so dangerous.

What power relations lurk in the scientific texts of the technology of physical fitness? The answer, I suggest, lies in the vision of life that those texts presuppose and help to reproduce. Revealing that vision entails seeing how the science and technology of physical fitness understands the body and its promise. What aspirations and limits to human potential does the technology of physical fitness hide in its texts on the body?

2

Theory of the Body: Technology, Puissance, Pouvoir

Although the capitalist order appears to be tolerant, it in fact has always controlled life through its expressive, sexual, emotional and affective aspects, constraining it to the dictates of its totalitarian organization based on exploitation, private property, male dominance, profit, and profitability. It exercises this control under all of its various guises: the family, schools, the work place, the army, rules, discourse. It unfailingly pursues its abject mission of castrating, oppressing, torturing, and mangling the body. All the better to inscribe its laws upon our flesh, to rivet into our unconscious its mechanisms for propagating slavery.

Guy Hocquenghem 1995, 260

In chapter 1, I suggested that scientific knowledge of the body is politically founded. But what of the body itself? What is the relationship between the body and society? Is the body a 'natural' entity engaged in social relations? Does it have a physical ontology apart from the social? Or is the body, its physicality, actually the product of sociocultural relations?[1]

My task in this chapter is to develop a theoretical framework that enables me to deconstruct (i.e., show the philosophy of the limit of) the politics of the body in the science and technology of physical fitness. The critical task is to develop a theory that shows how the body is available for social, cultural, and therefore political organization and to inquire into the general climate or spirit of the body in technological culture. How does the ontology of the body make it available to the politics of science and technology? Conversely, what is the ontology of technology that gives it access to the body? In other words, how does technology come to be insinuated in the body? I reiterate the questions of the philosophy of the limit from the Introduction above. How does technology construct a parergonal logic of the body that systematically includes and therefore excludes potentialities of the body? How does technology 'impose scarcity with a fundamental power of affirmation' (Foucault 1981, 73)? What dimensions of the body does technological discourse render second? And to what end?

What we therefore need here is a theory of the modern body that remains open to dimensions of the body's potential that have been made other – denied – by technology. To be faithful to this otherness, the theory needs to afford an identification with otherness that does not incorporate it into the theory. This is the negative dialectic crucial to the alterity of the philosophy of the limit and that informs the emotional dimension of this study as non-violent longing, which Adorno called a 'melancholy science.'

I begin with a discussion of technology, focusing on Heidegger's influential critique of modern technology as an aggressive way of being human and of making the world that ignores the intrinsic meaning of beings (for example, the earth, forests, animals, and human beings), in order to make them into useful resources. The parergonal logic of modern technology, I argue, goes to work on beings primarily, and in the worst circumstances *only*, in terms of their productive use-value, thus forgetting intrinsic, indeed spiritual, dimensions of Being-as-a-whole, dimensions that are essential to *well*-being. By the word 'spirit' I refer to the profound animating or generative quality of humans, animals, plants, the earth, and the universe. Such forgetfulness of spirit constitutes the parergonal logic of modernity, which, according to Heidegger, is therefore ultimately nihilistic. In other words, lurking beneath the 'progress' of modern technology is a terrible darkness, made all the darker by an increasingly pervasive cultural and socio-economic forgetting that there *are* qualities of light that lie within the darkness.

I contend that while the technological project forgets the spiritually enlightened dimensions of Being, those dimensions do not vanish altogether; the project renders them second to the work of technology and thus conceals them from the modern technological gaze. I try to explain the body in terms of its relationship to the meaning of Being and to the work of technology; I do so by reference to Deleuze and Guattari's (1983) theory of the body, specifically as it relates to discourse (134).

My theory of the body, especially in its application to the technology of physical fitness, serves the 'double function' of writing: 'to translate everything into assemblages and to dismantle the assemblages' (Deleuze and Guattari, quoted in Stivale 1998, 69). This theory of the body assembles a set of concepts (the task of this chapter) that we can use to pry apart the technology of physical fitness (chapter 3), with the aim of opening spaces for alternate ways of living (chapter 4). And so this book has a double constitution: while its earthbound 'lines of articulation' sediment the body in a theory that attempts to show how technology entraps the body, its 'lines of flight' open up a theoretical space that suggests the potential of practices that unleash the body's limitless, transcendent potency (Deleuze and Guattari 1987).

This chapter first considers the significance of the modern technological way of being. It then develops a theory of the bodily power that looks at its energy both as *puissance*, which is capable of transcendence, as powerful postmodern and non-Western concepts suggest, and as *pouvoir*, available to exploitation by modern technology.

Technology and the Body

I base my theory on Heidegger's (1938; 1954) account of technology, which articulates some of the fundamental dissatisfactions with modern life – namely, the insidious aggression and lack of genuine freedom – that also inspire the more explicit socially, economically, and politically predicated analyses of the other writers I use in this theory. The tyrannical aggression of the modern technological mode is manifestly evident in global degradation and in all-too-many cases of destruction of our planet's ecosphere; it is also apparent in the twentieth century's history of mass human extermination and the high-technological whirl of total war (Schell 2000); and in the human-made extinction of thousands of species of animals and plants, as well as the destruction of indigenous cultures. The destructive way that modern technological and patriarchal, white, Euro-American culture has dealt with the environment, under the guise of providing what is 'best' for 'man,' is, I suggest, also at work in the modern technological approach to the body; the techno-culture of physical fitness is a powerful manifestation of that approach. Indeed, perhaps if we can become more sensitive to the aggressive ways in which modernity deals with our *own* bodies, we may become more deeply aware of our aggression against the environment that surrounds us and the ecosphere that is essential to our life. More affirmatively, I suggest that Heidegger's concentration on the phenomenology of Being inspires a wonder that has affinities with the freeing potential for 'gaiety, ecstasy and dance' (Deleuze and Guattari 1987, 150), which are real possibilities, potential lines of flight, even within the aggression of modernity.

Heidegger's analysis of modernity focuses on its technology. Traditional social science and history have understood technology as the increasingly efficient use of energy, capital, and machinery in the process of economic production. David Krell (1977) summarizes that traditional view, saying that historians and social scientists locate the beginnings of modern technology

> in eighteenth-century England, where large coal deposits provide a source of energy for the production of steam, which in turn propels machinery in textile and other mills. But already at this relatively primitive stage of development the nexus of events becomes so complicated that nobody can neatly separate cause from effect ... Everything is jumbled together into inscrutable 'factors' – revolutionary discoveries in the natural sciences, detection and extraction of energy resources, invention of mechanical devices and chemical processes, availability of investment capital, improved means of transportation and communication, land enclosures, mechanization of agriculture, concentration of unskilled labour, a happy combination of this-worldly and other-worldly incentives – and the age of modern technology is off and running before anyone can catch his [sic] breath and raise a question. (284)

Technology is popularly understood as a matter of technique. High technology is the most sophisticated of techniques: supercomputers, genetic engineering, atomic energy, airliners, 'smart' bombs, and so on. But technology is more than a sophisticated ability to carry out tasks and further particular human ends. It is itself a cultural milieu that has profound effects on all aspects of earthly life. Michael Menser and Stanley Aronowitz (1996) describe the cultural dimension of technology in their introduction to *Technoscience and Cyberculture*: 'Technology is not simply a system to be deployed – as the US Army was deployed in the Persian Gulf; rather, it constitutes what we call "culture" itself ... Technologies, nature, and culture are all intertwined, not just in practice but *ontologically* [emphasis added]. Thus technologies are deployed, but they also employ and engage human beings and nature in such a manner that a continuity among the three arises that prevents any essential isolations of one from the other. That is, a subject cannot be defined simply as a human being. To be a subject is to be natural-cultural-technological; to be a social animal is to be techno-social ... Society, politics, perception, experience ... many of our most fundamental categories have been challenged or changed by technology' (21–2).

Menser and Aronowitz join Foucault and Rouse in seeing the essentially *productive* role of technology. Technology is not simply a tool for other projects. It is itself a project that produces realities: economic, political, social, cultural, psychological, biological, and spiritual. The *ontological* dimension of this production takes on profound significance when read in reference to Heidegger's understanding of the ontological essence of technology.

In contrast to the popular view, which sees technological life as the 'natural' result of 'discoveries' in the natural sciences and techniques of production, Heidegger suggests that technology is not the *product* of such discoveries, but a pervasive modern (Western) *disposition* towards beings that has engendered scientific and technical discovery or invention. Connecting this thought to Rouse's comments on science as a mode of engagement in the world, we could say that technology is a (practical) paradigm. (See the discussion of paradigms above in chapter 1). But this is not a paradigm simply in terms of technical procedures, familiarity with equipment and so forth. It is a practical paradigm in the more foundational sense of ways of disposing life and the world in general.

Heidegger says that the modern technological way of being human poses a great danger: it charts a destiny for human beings and the earth that is ultimately nihilistic. His concern is not with the particularities of various technologies (the dangers of nuclear technology, for instance), but with the ultimate journey that the modern technological mode charts for people and the planet. Heidegger asks about the *essence* of modern technology. In posing such a question he suggests that modern technology is not just a medium taken up by various human projects; it has its own impetus. That impetus is is essence.

Many people participating in recent debates in the human sciences consider the word 'essence' problematic. They conceive that which is essential as the politically conservative opposite of that which more radical perspectives see as socially constructed and therefore alterable. They see an essence as ahistorical, natural, immutable. One essentialist understanding of gender, for instance, conceives women as 'naturally' the caretakers of men and children – a transhistorical aspect of human 'nature.' Conversely, Heidegger's understanding of essence (in German he uses the word *Wesen*) is profoundly historical. For him, it means the manner in which things come to presence, the way in which they are realized. It is the historical *manner* by which things become the way they are and that therefore sets what they become. In this sense, essences, as manners of becoming, chart historical destinies. If, for instance, the essence of womanhood in a patriarchal system is subservience to the mastery of men, then the destiny of those people who are made women in such a system is very likely to be slavery. Fortunately, it is sometimes possible, given the right historical circumstances, to change destiny by changing the manner of becoming. That is, if we can change our essence, we can change how we are. This is not easy. Critical social constructionists dislike talk of essences because they see it positing an oppressive stasis to social categories that cannot be overcome. My appropriation of Heidegger's understanding of essence, in contrast, understands it as the very nexus of the dynamic temporality by which things happen.

What then is the essence of modern technology? Departing from the traditional understanding, Heidegger (1954) says that the essence of 'technology is nothing technological' (317) – not mechanical inventions, chemical manipulations, advanced transportation, communication, and the like; these are but the products of technology. The essence of technology is the way in which it reveals or produces beings. *Modern* technology, he says, does so by challenging them to be revealed as 'standing-reserve' (298) – something ordered to be used for something else, or a resource. The essence of technology is manifest in this way of revealing beings – the paradigm realizes beings as resources. And modern technology is unlike ancient Greek technology, for instance, in which *techne* is a form of *poiesis*, a compassionate bringing forth of what is there (291–3). Modern technology, in contrast, is aggressive; it reveals things according to projects that are external to them. An example might help. The ancient Greek understanding of sculpture was that the sculptor helped the statue concealed in the marble to emerge from the marble; it was a careful bringing forth of what was there – *poiesis*, an original uncovering. Modern technology takes what is there in its own way and turns it into something else, a resource for some project. It sees a forest, for example, as nothing but a source of materials for the pulp and paper industry; it turns it aggressively into something else. This modern way does reveal the forest in one aspect – as a resource. It ignores, even undermines, the other ways in which a forest reveals itself – as a home for animals, a mysterious place, something in its own right. The word 'resource' comes from the Latin root *surgere*, which means 'to rise'; the prefix 're' means 'again.' Originally the forest is simply there, arising, as it were on its own terms, useless to industry. When re-sourced, it arises again, not as simply there, but as useful to industry. And such re-sourcing, as clear-cut logging attests, is no small intervention into what was originally simply there, un-dis-covered as something useful to humans.

Even humans become resources: most large public and private enterprises, such as my university (the University of Toronto) no longer have personnel departments – they are now departments of human resources; children are frequently called a nation's greatest resource! Students work hard at school in order to realize themselves as excellent resources in a competitive labour market. The Canadian government has a ministry of human resources that has a branch called 'Human Resource Development Canada,' which conducts research and develops policies for the management of 'human resource capital.' As part of its work it maintains an enormous, computerized database that co-ordinates information on all Canadian citizens, so that it can better develop their capital potential. Such re-sourcing of human being is sinister because, marshalled as a resource, human essence (our realization) is our use-value or exchange-value.[2]

Harold Alderman (1978) develops Heidegger's analysis of technology as a disposition towards beings that marshals them as resources, adding that where there are resources there also are waste products (46–7). He takes the example of mining, which secures its resources in a discriminating and decisive way. Strip mining is the most blatant example – tearing up the earth and casting off all but the ore that it seeks. Indeed, advanced technology disposes of beings precisely by determining what is a resource and what is a waste product. The problems with this attitude towards the environment are now well known (see Foltz 1995; Llewellyn 1991; 1993). And in the North American 'human resource sector' in the corporate downsizing of the 1990s, more and more working-class people lost their (dubious) status as resources and became waste products in the increasingly efficient production of wealth that becomes the preserve of ever fewer and fewer people (Greenspon 1996; Tough 1996). By the turn of the century, this had led to the distinct polarization of resource rich and poor in the United States, Canada, and Britain.

Heidegger postulates a metaphysical background for modern technology, a metaphysics that is also the background for modern science. Many assume that modern technology has been made possible by the advances of modern science. Heidegger says that a more fundamental historical shift lies at the heart of the modernity of both science and technology. This is the historical shift in which man [sic] becomes the measure of all things.

Before describing this historical shift, I offer a few words on Heidegger's use of the word 'man:' It could be argued that Heidegger uses the word 'man' rather than 'humanity,' because he is reproducing the historical sexist practice of using the word 'man' to represent both men and women, showing insensitivity, unawareness, or even a wilful desire to obliterate the different ways in which women and men may relate to the world in which they find and create themselves. One can, however, read Heidegger's use of that common form, applied to the aggressiveness of modern technology, as a gendered sensitivity to the domineering, patriarchal nature of the modern technological project. He chose his words carefully when signifying the beings commonly called humans – in *Being and Time* (1927) he uses the gender-neutral *Dasein*, by which he means openness to being, rather than 'man' or 'human,' which he finds carry too much metaphysical baggage. When he speaks of 'man the technologist,' one can read not only long-standing metaphysical traditions, but also long-standing patriarchal gendered traditions. Heidegger's account of technology *is* androcentric; but then, the history of modern technology is also androcentric – originally, and still predominantly, produced by European, North American, and Asian men (and not all of them at that), with women in ancillary roles. Indeed, Heidegger deals *only* with those philosophical, scientific, poetic, and fine art texts that men have produced. Thus we can read him literally: he is describing a masculine tradition in Western culture. And as feminist philosophers of science have argued, the domineering spirit of Western science and technology is patriarchal (Bleier 1984; Ginzberg 1989; Haraway 1988; Harding 1986; Hubbard 1989; 1990; Keller 1989; 1992; Longino 1989; Rosser 1990). While Heidegger does not thematize gender, his critique of technology as an aggressive, domineering relationship to beings is also a well-trodden feminist critique of patriarchy. While women, like men, have been included in the technological project (mostly to their peril), it is men who have been largely responsible for it.[3] In order to keep in mind the androcentric foundations of modern technology, I will use the word 'man' as I develop the technological basis of this theory of the body in the next few paragraphs. Because I do not want to suggest that women are not part of the project, because certainly many now are, I generally use the word 'human.'

Let us return to the historical shift that renders man the measure of all things. Heidegger says that everything that is for man, or at least everything that matters, is what can be represented by man to himself. In this, man has become the *hupkeimenon* – i.e., that which becomes the foundation of all that is made present. For Plato, the *hupkeimenon* was the *eidos*; for Aristotle, actuality. For the Christian church the *hupkeimenon* was God as revealed in sacred scriptures and sacraments. With Descartes, whose *cogito ergo sum* announces for Heidegger the philosophical centre of modernity, the *hupokeimenon* is the subjectivity of man.[4] 'I think, therefore I am.' When man becomes *hupokeimenon*, he takes considerable power over what he beholds.

Heidegger believes that while 'man as the measure of all things' reaches its fullest philosophical expression in Descartes and the modern projects of science and technology, it originates in the metaphysical tradition that began in fifth-century (BCE) Greece, when an appreciation of the essential, mysterious, *hidden* power of nature that is celebrated in Anaximander, Parmenides, and Heraclitus gradually gives way to the attitude that every aspect of nature is available to the inspecting, knowing, anthropocentric, *revealing* power of man (Sheehan 1981, 540). This is the far-reaching Western patriarchal cultural tradition that Derrida and others have called phallogocentrism. In his exposition of the North American Native philosophy on the place of human beings in the life of the earth, Calvin Luther Martin (1999) also comments on the advent of this anthropocentrism. He gives it a much longer history, however, saying that it inheres in the development of agriculture, which marks the Neolithic moment: 'With the advent of the Neolithic plants and animals were stripped of their *will* and *permission* and forced to submit to a schedule that suited one mathematical mammal's sense of thrift' (8). This occurred at different times in different places. Martin says that archaeologists suggest the earliest was some seven thousand to ten thousand years ago, and it is an event that continues in those corners of the world that still engage in hunter-gatherer culture in the encroaching shadow of modern global capitalism.

The Hebrew book of Genesis attempts to justify this logic of domination in its first creation myth: 'God said, "Let us make man in our own image, in the likeness of ourselves, and let them be masters of the fish of the sea, the birds of heaven, the cattle, all the wild animals and all the creatures that creep along the ground"' (Genesis 1:26, *The New Jerusalem Bible*). As I argue in the next chapter, logics of domination and sovereignty are essential to the Judaeo-Christian traditions of subject formation, logics that continue in an ironically inverted fashion in modern subjectivity, in which the sovereignty of man replaces the sovereignty of God. And as Trish Glazebrook (in press) suggests in an article on Heidegger and ecofeminism, this anthropocentrism is gendered; indeed, some have argued that anthropocentrism is actually androcentrism (Kheel 1988; 1990; Spretnak 1990; Zimmerman 1987).

Central to this subjectivity is the power of projecting onto things conceptual frameworks for knowing them in advance of empirical encounters with them. For the modern *scientific* subject, this is a matter of seeing things in their objectness, by which Heidegger means their calculability. All that is can be pictured on a measurable grid of linear time and space. Calculability establishes the parergonal logic of science. In 'Modern Science, Metaphysics and Mathematics' (1962), Heidegger points out that in this grid, space and time are not specific. He speaks of Newton's doctrine of motion: 'Every body left to itself moves uniformly in a straight line.' The crucial word here is *every* body. Any sense of things moving from themselves because of their own nature is removed here, rendered second by the parergonal logic that sees *every* body as being essentially the same. (Heidegger contrasts this with Aristotle's conception of bodies moving according to their nature – for example, heavenly bodies moving up and earthly bodies moving down.) For the modern scientific subject, everything worth thinking about can be represented in this way; no account needs to be made of the particular and inherent nature of things, of the way in which they may appear from themselves. Modern science, Heidegger says, projects onto beings this fundamental (and narrow) notion of their being.

Projection is what Heidegger means by mathematics, *ta mathemata*, what we know in advance of the experience of beings, such as their calculability in time and space and their resourcefulness within prede-

termined systems of use-value. From the perspective of the philosophy of the limit, then, the conceptual framework of *ta mathemata* institutes the logic of parergonality, of what the system includes. So calculated, beings become objects for the modern scientific subject and hence
resources for social, economic, and political projects. Seeing things in
their calculability makes them more easily available for human projects;
it sets forth a conceptual framework for the manipulation of things to
human ends. This capacity to deal with everything with the working
assumption that they are there for the human subject increases substantially the human capacity for control of what is there. Deference to
otherness (alterity) disappears, except where there is detectable resistance by that which is other. And where science encounters resistance,
rather than pursuing paths of alterity, it usually looks for new anthropocentric concepts that are capable of incorporating and therefore erasing otherness and undermining the resistance of that which had frus-
trated the scientific gaze.

Objects, in the above sense, are only theoretical. Ostensibly, it is
possible to conceive of beings in their objectness and still allow that
they may appear in ways that are not calculable or resourceful. This
would be a matter of seeing beings as objects as but one concept of
them, one that may be helpful, but that could also be problematic. The
great danger lies in not distinguishing between the *conception* of beings as objects and the treatment of them as if that is what they are
essentially – that is, only as represented to man as objects for scientific
calculation and technological resourcing. In 'The Age of the World
Picture,' Heidegger (1938) suggests that what happens in the modern
age is that the picture of beings as calculable objects comes to limit the
sense of what can emerge. In this sense the picturing representation is
supreme; what is is what man represents to himself. That picturing
Heidegger calls *Gestell* (enframing), the setting of a framework for the
possibilities of reality. That which does not appear in the framework
either does not matter or, more violently, is erased from meaningful
existence in a framework that sees only that which is potentially useful as a resource. Obviously, there is significant affinity between
Heidegger's concept of the limiting work of framework and Drucilla
Cornell's philosophy of the limit, in which the parergonal logic is the
enframing of resourcefulness and secondness is all that is 'useless' to,
or a waste product of, the project.

Science serves technology by offering sophisticated representations
of beings as objects. Technological man then takes that objective repre-

sentation and forgets that he has made the objects reveals beings as only resources. Heidegger says that the great danger comes when what is revealed is revealed *exclusively* as a resource. In this exclusivity there is no other potential: the only revelation of human being is as resource-full. This means that our essence (our manner of becoming) is determined by the social, cultural, political, and economic structures that set its use-value. The value of human life becomes contingent on its coherence with the finite, economic, calculative logic of usefulness and productivity. The meaning of human being is defined extrinsically.

This amounts to a failure to appreciate and consequently to care for the unfathomable meaning intrinsic to the mystery of Being itself. The danger here is that modern technological human beings miss the opportunity to live fully in the wonder and profound freedom of Being. But this is not just a matter of missing an opportunity for some individual experience of mystery, rapture, or insight. For this fundamental, historical lack of appreciation of Being brings with it an aggressive kind of uncaring, through which we order not only our individual selves but also our fellow human and other beings in a way that precludes any other revelation – it becomes a productive, dominating force. John Caputo (1986) remarks: 'The danger ... is that the essence of man and of truth will be perverted once for all, that the grip of the *Gestell* will be unbreakable, that the world-night will grow darker' (xviii). In 'Science and Reflection,' Heidegger (1953) invokes the metaphors of light and darkness, saying that our modern way has cast a shadow over the light of Being. By continuing to live in such a shadow, without reflecting on the light that is withheld by it, we fail to fulfil our most fundamental responsibilities as beings who have the capacity to care for the way in which we and our fellow beings, both human and otherwise, are realized. As ecofeminists and deep ecologists have argued, the dark power of anthropocentric thought and practice has brought us to an ecological crisis that may now be a path of inevitable, and perhaps even total, destruction of life on this planet (Gottlieb 1996).

The great, indeed promising irony secreted in the dangers of the technological paradigm is that while modern technology reveals beings as mere resources, as a mode of revealing, it is still a becoming. And in that *energy of becoming* there is hope, albeit remote. In an interestingly deconstructive vein, Heidegger (1954b) defines freedom in 'The Question Concerning Technology' as follows: 'Freedom is that which conceals in a way that opens to light, in whose lighting shimmers that veil that hides the essential occurrence of all truth and lets the veil appear as what veils' (306). If we become aware of technology as a domineering, marshalling force and attend not to the what (i.e., the technical things produced in technology) but to the how of its revelation (i.e., marshalling our essence, re-sourcing our reality), we can find freedom from technological destiny: 'For man becomes truly free only insofar as he belongs to the realm of destining and so becomes one who listens, *though not one who simply obeys*' (306, emphasis added).

Listening to our technological essence in order to disobey its profoundly limiting framework is perhaps the key to challenging what we are becoming. It may be the cipher that can change our destiny. Indeed, the point of this book is to listen to one particular manifestation of modern technology – physical fitness – in order to detect what we are becoming, thus fostering the remote hope that there is still a chance to sway our destiny.

Modern technology grounds human possibilities in the economics and logics of resource management. Where it is most powerful, it *demands* that people become good resources; it restricts the possibilities for human becoming to the destiny of extrinsic usefulness. Increasingly, this has become the impetus of formal education: to train young people as good resources for the economic system. In the next chapter I suggest that physical education based in the technology of physical fitness demands the subordination of human physical, indeed *erotic* potential to the logic and economics of bodily resource management. In the pages below, I suggest that the demands of resource management foreclose on the potential for freedom and therefore for meaningful encounter with truth. Keeping in mind Heidegger's thought: 'The essence of truth is freedom ... Freedom lets beings be the beings they are' (1961), I argue that modern technology, as the preeminent ground for being in the modern world, restricts significantly the cultural imagination of the possibilities of true freedom. And as Foucault, Turner, and many others have argued at length, the body is *the* site for the modern production of human freedom and constraint.

Puissance

What is the essence of the body? What about its essence makes it available as a resource? How is it thus configured? What is rendered second when the body is resourced?

I now give Heidegger's philosophy on the resourcing of beings a more explicitly political and embodied twist by placing in the context of power his notion of 'essence' as the manner of realization and resourcing as an aggressive marshalling of the actuality of the body. I invoke two senses of power under two French signs: *puissance* and *pouvoir*. These are words that Deleuze and Guattari use to signify two different kinds of power (Massumi 1992, xvii).[5] Massumi defines them succinctly as follows: '*Puissance* refers to a range of potential. It has been defined by Deleuze as a "capacity for existence," "a capacity to affect or be affected" [which refers not only to emotion, but to the augmentation or diminution of the body's capacity to act], a capacity to multiply connections that may be realized by a given "body" to varying degrees in different situations ... It is used in French translation of Nietzsche's "will to power." ... The authors use *pouvoir* in a sense very close to Foucault's, as an instituted and reproducible relation of force, a selective concretization of potential' (xvii).[6]

For ease of explication, I begin by discussing puissance and pouvoir separately for the most part, although, as we see below, they need to be understood in reference to each other. In practice they work or play dynamically, producing the energy that is modern, phallogocentric life.[7] My theory of the body is not a transhistorical, pan-cultural theory – it attempts to account for the life of those bodies that are produced in the shadow of technological modernity, a force that is historically white, patriarchal, capitalist, and Euro-American, which is encroaching in variable and uneven ways around the world. This is, then, a theory of the modern body as dynamic, concentrating on the energy produced in the interplay of puissance and pouvoir in modern techno-culture. This theory reconceptualizes, as itself a manifestation of pouvoir, the dominant concept of the body as an individual, biological object that occupies a discrete space–time continuum organized along functional, systematic lines (which is how the natural sciences see and represent the body).

Here is a synopsis of the theory. Pouvoir sets about re-sourcing elements of puissance, which give life to pouvoir, thus making embodied cultural capital, which circulates in the economics of production, consumption, and debris. This re-sourcing and marketing constitute a dynamic, historical process that, for a host of reasons and under an infinite number of different circumstances, not only uses up but also lays waste and fortunately sometimes overlooks vast 'regions' of puissance – i.e., secondness, in the logic of parergonality.

This theory of the body is not of course exhaustive; I offer it as a tool to understand the fate of the body in modern technology. Puissance, as I attempt to explain, is infinite and thus eludes any identity of sign and signified. I present my words on puissance not as adequate representations of this reality, but as an invitation for the reader to reflect on its actuality or at least potential in her or his own experience. And pouvoir has many dimensions that may or may not intersect with the technological project that I am trying to show. Moreover, because mine is not a history project, this is not an account of the many processes that brought the technological body to pass. Finally, and most important, my theory of puissance and pouvoir could be mistaken as a constitutional polarity (puissance = good, pouvoir = bad). Puissance is not the opposite of pouvoir; it is a *resource* for the governmentality (Foucault 1979; 1980b; 1988) of pouvoir. Pouvoir has no power without puissance, whereas puissance does have power without pouvoir.

I begin with the body's essence. Above I contrasted Heidegger's understanding of essence with the essentialism that has been criticized by social constructionists who have criticized it for imposing an imperial, defining, and limiting gaze on the potential for experience. 'Essence,' as Heidegger uses it, and as I am taking it up, need not necessarily denote an imperial gaze.[8] 'Imperial essentialism,' if you will, is a social construction that fills human being with cultural content based in systems for the organization of life, such as gender, sexuality, race, and technology. 'Essence,' in that sense, is supposed to determine *what* (in terms of content) people fundamentally are, how they should be interpreted, and the social context in which their lives should unfold. There is, however, another essential dimension that is ontologically prior to the *whatness of being* and pertains to the life-giving power (puissance) of *being at all*. This power is essential to all beings (which, of course, includes human beings); it is the power of coming to presence, the productive power of realization – in Deleuze's definition of puissance, above, it would be the capacity to exist, the capacity to affect and be affected.[9]

But the puissance of coming to presence is not just 'to be (or exist), in the sense of a potential that may or may not be actualized; it is the urgent, eventful process of presen*cing*. To be emphasized here is *pro-cess*' (Sheehan 1981, 536): the process of be-ing that makes possible the presencing of cultural content. And in that process of coming to presence lies the potential both to construct and to deconstruct cultural content (whatness). The ethical and political problems that may be associated with essence as coming to presence lie not in being as coming to presence as such, but in *ways* of coming to presence – more specifically, the harmful ways in which socio-cultural forces compel beings to come to presence, or the way historical discourses produce their essence.

I develop the concept of puissance in terms of four processes that lead to what the Buddhists term 'emptiness.' This progression – through movement, to reflection, thence to desire, and beyond that to emptiness – opens enormous possibilities. Adapting Robert Glass's (1995) synthesis of postmodern, quantum mechanical, and Buddhist thought, I then apply powerful concepts – the Body without Organs, One Bright Pearl, the Body of Reality, and Indra's Net, as well as particle and wave theories of light – to consider the freedom that flows from emptiness and finally the embodying of emptiness.

Movement

The process by which the living body comes to presence is movement. If there is no movement, there is no life. Thomas Sheehan (1981) points out that Heidegger similarly understood *being itself* as movement: 'The unifying topic [of Heidegger's] program was, from first to last, movement' (539). Heidegger sought to address the Western tradition's lack of appreciation of movement, indeed its incessant attempt to get some control over being by bringing some stasis to its movement – Sheehan refers to this as the 'hypostatization of being.'[10] In that context, Heidegger questioned the foundations of our experience of 'reality.' He said that we have inherited a phenomenological mode of experience from the Greeks, evidenced from Homer to Aristotle, which is that we experience things analogically, as they show themselves '*as* something meaningful' (Sheehan 1983, 137). In Western experience, 'man can deal with entities only insofar as they appear *as* such and so' (138, emphasis added). This is the *logos:* an openness to being that gathers together and lays before us what is there (Heidegger 1975), in the form of a hermeneutic circle that allows it to appear in the analogies of meaning structures.

An example based in my earlier discussion of technology may help. The *logos* of modern technology is an openness to the being of entities that understands them already as potential resources/waste products. Here is the openness that one finds in an enclosure. The forest thus comes to presence for the technological forester *as* a resource – such an appearance of the forest comes from the forester's education and training in the logos of modern forest management. Technology is a logos. Similarly, there are *logoi* of gender and race that give gendered and raced meaning to the appearance of people. Phallocentrism is the logos that renders meaningful reality in the structure, logic, and desire of the dominating and space-occupying phallic enterprise: the conquering will-to-power of the Western patriarchal tradition. But there is a logos that goes beyond technology, race, and gender – an openness to being that makes be-ing itself meaningful. It is a particularly powerful logos in so far as it gives meaning that does not 'add up to a system of belief or an architecture of propositions that you either enter or you don't, but instead pack[s] a potential in the way a crowbar in a willing hand evokes an energy of prying' (Massumi 1992, 8).

Heidegger says that what makes being meaningful is time. In *Being and Time* (1927), he describes how Dasein's authentic appreciation of its own death makes time palpable and gives being a truly urgent meaningfulness. There, the contemplation of one's own death as the negation of one's presence brings to one a shattering awareness and appreciation of presence. In his much-discussed and mostly-misunderstood 'turn' *(Kehre)* (Sheehan 1981, 539), Heidegger articulates the logos of being not as the world-shattering appreciation of presence that sings in the shadow of its own negation, the onset of absence that is death, but as the revelation (*aletheia* – more accurately: unconcealment) of absence as the fountain of presence as it is manifest in the *event* of movement, which Heidegger (1972) calls *Ereignis* and that I attempt to explain below. This is, I think, a major shift in thinking, away from the philosophy of ultimate lack that fuels the existential crisis of facing death. Here, presence and absence become a powerful synergy that expresses the awe-full power of being in the wonderful event of movement, which is the essence of being.

The logos of being, the openness to being that gathers together what is there so that its be-ing is meaningful, is the logos that gathers together the relations of absence and presence as *movement*. The body appears in the logos, the meaningfulness, of movement. My theory of the body is thus a theory of its essences as revealed in the logos of its movements – puissance and pouvoir. The logos of puissance reveals the meaning of the body as motile being, as the profound, eventful gift manifest in life itself. The logos of pouvoir reveals the meaning of the moving body as socio-culturally known, governed, and produced.

Heidegger draws his understanding of being as movement from Aristotle, saying that it is the play of presence and absence: 'For Aristotle, Heidegger points out, all natural entities are kinetic in an ontological way: their *kinesis* is their very being. A moving entity is one that does not fully appear (is not completely present) and yet does appear precisely in its incompleteness. We understand a plant as a plant, for example, only by knowing that its presence is fraught with absentiality: a not yet and no longer, a coming into and a going from presence. Such relative absentiality is what makes the entity *be* the moving entity it is. Therefore, to really know a natural thing means to keep present to mind not only the present entity but also the *presence of the absentiality* that makes it kinetic. The presence-of-its-absentiality (or its privative presence) is the moving entity's being-structure' (Sheehan 1981, 537).

More appropriate to a theory of the body than the observation of the movement of plants is the movement of the body. David Michael Levin (1985) says: 'The field of our motility is the *layout* [*logos*] of a field of Being: it is how Being manifests, how Being presences, in relation to our motility' (94). The puissance of the body is its being, its coming to presence, its essence as movement. In contrast to Sheehan, who discerns presence and absence in movement from a relatively disengaged visual perception of the movement of 'other' objects (what we know about plants because we have seen them grow), I attempt to explicate the relations of absence and presence by reflecting on the immediacy, the intensity of the experience of moving.

Reflection

Reflection (*Besinnung*) is the methodological heart of Heidegger's appreciation of being and movement (Heidegger 1927; 1953; 1954a; 1954b; 1954c; 1966; 1972). 'Reflection' (*Besinnung*) is an experience that is different from representational thinking, for which Heidegger uses the word *vorstellen*, which suggests the mind's observing itself (Heidegger 1953, 156, translator's note). Reflection, in contrast, is a deliberative recollection that considers the sense (*Sinn*) or meaning of the *passage* of the event of being. Reflection opens us to the spirit of the event of being as actualizing presencing rather than as providing an object-ive re-presentation of what happened. There is no distance in reflection.

Reflection occurs in meditative thinking, which is very much unlike the authoritative ways of thinking in Western culture, which are dominating and calculative, realized most fully in the re-presentational, re-sourcing power of modern technology. The power of reflection is not high-flying theorizing, as in the work of high-end modern physics or, in the complexities of deconstruction theory or other postmodern currents. The power of reflection comes from meditating on what is closest to us. 'It is enough to dwell on what lies close and meditate on what is closest; upon that which concerns us, each one of us, here and now; *here*, on this patch of home ground; *now* in the present hour of history' (Heidegger 1966, 47).

I suggest that what is closest to each of us, here and now, is our own be-ing, the movement that is the life which becomes present in each breath, with each heartbeat. The closest thing to me is the immediate space, or opening, that allows me to be or, more accurately, to become. This 'space' is the beneficence that Heidegger refers to in *On Time and Being* (1972) as the eventful 'Giving' of Be-*ing*: 'To think Being explicitly requires us to relinquish Being as the ground of be-ings in favor [*sic*] of the giving which prevails concealed in uncon-cealment, that is in favor [*sic*] of the It gives. As the gift of this It gives, Being belongs to giving. As a gift, Being is not expelled from giving. Being, presencing is transmuted. As allowing-to-presence, it belongs to unconcealing: as the gift of unconcealing it is retained in the giving. Being *is* not. There is, It gives Being as the unconcealing; as the gift of unconcealing it is retained in the giving. Being *is* not. There is, It gives Being as the unconcealing of presencing' (6).

By meditating on the gift of our coming to presence, which is the nearest of all nears, we make reflection possible. Reflection arises in the resolve to attend to the event of be-ing as movement (Ereignis); it is akin to dwelling in and appreciating the wonder of the journey of life, which is just as much the passage from moment into moment as it is the passage from youth into old age, and perhaps even more so. Reflection brings us into the midst of the event that Frederick Turner (8) calls 'the joy of full presence' and that Calvin Luther Martin (1999, 31) says is 'the holiness of beauty.' As such, reflection is the opposite of calculative explanations of what happened to one: absent father and overbearing mother, unresolved Oedipus complex, sexual abuse in childhood, co-dependence, psycho-chemical imbalance, and so on.

Reflection, says Heidegger (1953), 'is more than a mere making conscious of something. We do not yet have reflection when we have only consciousness. Reflection is more. It is calm, self-possessed surrender to that which is worthy of questioning. Through reflection, so understood, we actually arrive at the place where, without having experienced it and without having seen penetratingly into it, we have long been sojourning. In reflection we gain access to a place from out of which there first opens the space traversed at any given time by all our doing and leaving undone' (180). In 'On the Way to *Ereignis*,' Sheehan (1983) says: 'Only in resolve does one enter *Ereignis*; only by taking up personally one's own movement does one authentically discover the movement that is being itself. The meaning of being, as Richardson has said, is not a doctrine to be learned but a risk to be taken. And if one does not take that risk, Heidegger told his students, "all talk and listening is in vain"' (163).

Such reflection on one's own movements poses a serious risk to the organization of the socially produced human self (the subject of pouvoir). Caputo (1986) writes: 'Wakefulness does not emancipate us *from* the oblivion, but *to* it' (xxiii). As I try to show below, intense awareness of movement deconstructs the self as such and reveals a non-selfish dimension. David Michael Levin (1987) has argued the same point, making explicit connections between Heidegger and some of the foundational traditions of Buddhism in the concept *mudra* – a way of embodiment that manifests Buddhist enlightenment: 'The importance of *mudra* for our access to this bodily wisdom lies in the fact that we are situated in a field that breaks down our ego-structured encapsulations and opens us up to the being of other sentient natures. Thus, *mudra* contributes to our self-development by anchoring our life in the compassion of a transpersonal field' (246).

Deleuze and Guattari describe engagement in plateaus of intensity that free the body of limiting discursive imperatives such as the delineated, discrete self, which is constructed/organized (pouvoir) in discourses such as gender, race, and technology. The intensity of movement reveals a dimension and potential for the body that is not externally organized (the subject of pouvoir); it is rather a de-organized (deterritorialized) Body without Organs (which Deleuze and Guattari [1987] signify with 'BwO') that is free. Agreeing that engaging in the intensities of the moving body poses risks, they say: 'And how necessary caution is, the art of dosages, since overdose is a danger. You don't do it with a sledgehammer, you use a very fine file. You invent self-destructions that have nothing to do with the death drive. Dismantling the organism has never meant killing yourself, but rather opening the body to connections that presuppose an entire assem-

blage, circuits, conjunctions, levels and thresholds, passages and distributions of intensity, and territories and deterritorializations measured with the craft of a surveyor' (160).

But with this danger comes the potential for experiments with freedom, a freedom that goes beyond the self. Levin (1985) observes: 'As
we let go of the ego-logical, ego-centric structure which typically characterizes our present experience of motility in its personal–interpersonal field, going (as it were) *beneath* it in an attempt to make contact
with our more primordial attunement by Being as a whole, what we
encounter, along the way, is a *prepersonal* and, in fact a *transpersonal*
dimension; and our contact with the motivating energies at work in
this dimension of our experiential motility field can have profoundly
therapeutic effects, radically transforming our experience, for example,
of the very *ground* of interpersonal solicitude' (97).

Crucial to the following explication of the moving body is the potential that it affords for profoundly ecological, *collective,* and transcendental rather than individual, anomic, ways of finding meaning
and of living. Heidegger (1975), in his essay on Heraclitus's saying
(Fragment 50) on the Logos – 'Listening not to me but to the Logos, it
is wise to agree that all things are one' – says that openness to being
reveals the essential connectedness of our existence. Deleuze and
Guattari point to this, above, suggesting that the body be opened to
'connections that presuppose an entire assemblage, circuits, conjunctions, levels and thresholds, passages and distributions of intensity.'
Merleau-Ponty (1962) refers to this collectivity as 'flesh,' a 'prepersonal
tradition,' that *is* the body: 'My personal existence must be the re-
sumption of a prepersonal tradition. There is , therefore, another subject beneath me, for whom a world exists before I am here, and who
marks out my place in it. This captive or natural spirit is my body ... a
communication with the world more ancient than thought' (254). Calvin
Luther Martin (1999), commenting on the North American Native appreciation of humans' profound kinship with all living beings, calls
this the 'Common Self' – the beauty and power of the deepest meaning of kinship. To live in that dimension of profound relatedness, he
says, 'is to become a truly genuine person' (40). For Deleuze and
Guattari, this prepersonal 'tradition' is the Body without Organs (BwO),
a dimension of the body that is always already there, but which is for
the most part already appropriated and bound by discourses that would
deny its essential transcendent collectivity, by reining in the freedom
of its movements. Similarly, Heidegger (1953): '[We] arrive at the place

where, without having experienced it and without having seen penetratingly into it, we have long been sojourning. In reflection we gain access to a place from out of which there first opens the space traversed at any given time by all our doing and leaving undone' (180).

Desire

Deleuze and Guattari (1987) ask: 'How Do You Make Yourself a Body without Organs?' And they answer:

> At any rate, you have one (or several). It's not so much that it preexists or comes ready-made, although in certain respects it is preexistent. At any rate, you make one, you can't desire without making one. And it awaits you; it is an inevitable exercise or experimentation, already accomplished the moment you undertake it, unaccomplished as long as you don't. This is not reassuring, because you can botch it. Or it can be terrifying, and lead you to your death ... It is not at all a notion or a concept but a practice, a set of practices. You never reach the Body without Organs, you can't reach it, you are forever attaining it, it is a limit. People ask, So what is this BwO? – But you are already on it, scurrying like a vermin, groping like a blind person, or running like a lunatic desert traveller and nomad of the steppes. On it we sleep, live our waking lives, fight – fight and are fought – seek our place, experience untold happiness and fabulous defeats; on it we penetrate and are penetrated; on it we love. (150–1)

Here, as in Heidegger, there is a call to attend to the event of our coming to presence, of appreciating it as a happening, a journey, under way, a practice, fraught with presence and absence, more than individual, never completely revealed, and risky. Heidegger understands this coming to presence as the movement of being; in the movements of individual human beings, the movement of being as whole is mysteriously manifest. Using the somewhat sexier language of desire, Deleuze and Guattari conceptualize the power of being explicitly as embodiment: they speak of the productive power of desire that takes place in the holism of the BwO. For Deleuze and Guattari, desire is not a means to an end – the desire for sex in order to procreate, the desire for food in order to sustain life, the desire for social networks in order to support and strengthen the ego, the desire for physical exercise to calm one's nerves, the desire for money to buy desired stuff. Desire is not a lack of something else, a hole that needs to be filled. Desire, they say, is a productive force, and 'the real is the end product' (1983, 26). It is the potency of becoming or actualizing, a potency so intense that it seeks no culmination or resolution. Indeed the culmination of desire is an *a posteriori* lack of desire, desire's undoing. Desire is productive affirmation. In *Anti-Oedipus*, Deleuze and Guattari (1983) refer to the desiring body as the 'desiring machine' – they mean the word 'machine' to evoke the power of machines to produce, rather than the mechanical servitude to owners and systems that use them. They say: 'It is precisely to underline the artificial "constructivist" nature of desire that we defined it as "machinic," which is to say articulated with the most actual, the most "urgent" machinic types' (Stivale 1998, 99).

What does the desiring machine produce? Flows of desire – movement. Crucial to this sensibility of the desiring body is its anti-stasis: it is eventful, productive, affecting. In *A Thousand Plateaus*, Deleuze and Guattari (1987) define desire as 'a process of production without reference to any exterior agency' (154). What is important here is the notion of desire as a process, or movement. Desire is the fundamental, productive, moving process by which the body is. In as much as Deleuze and Guattari eschew foundational philosophy, sensing in it a dictatorial restriction on whatever follows, they do posit the puissance of desire as an energy that lives in some relationship to other kinds of energy – their particular interest is the energy of capitalism and the ways in which it shapes the flows of desire. There is an essential energy about desire that *could* be free of the dictates of culture – an energy that capitalism seeks to harness (re-source/*Gestell*). As such, desire is immensely valuable to capitalist culture, social organization, and economics. Certainly, as Foucault and others have convincingly argued, it is the organization of desire that produces modern culture, society, and economics. The *Capitalism and Schizophrenia* books (Deleuze and Guattari, 1983; 1987) tell the story of the fate of desire under capitalism.

In their focus on dynamic processes of production, Deleuze and Guattari share thematic focus with Heidegger, who articulates his concerns under the sign of 'being.' Deleuze and Guattari, however, barely mention Heidegger,[11] and explicitly distance their own work from ontological philosophy: Massumi (1992) points out: 'To avoid philosophical baggage, they are more likely to say that a thing is "actual" than that it "exists." To drive it home that actuality is dynamic they use the word "becoming" in place of "being." A thing's actuality is its duration as a process – of genesis and annihilation, of movement across thresholds and toward a limit' (37). The 'philosophical baggage' that is supposed to tag along with discussions of being is that 'being' represents a reified entrapment of desire in transhistorical form, an oppressive 'state' that we have inherited from the Greeks. Talk of being is nothing more than an expression of a pathetic nostalgia for the security of ancient wisdom, the ontotheology of the Western tradition (Taylor 1987), the world of the living dead.

But it would be a great waste of Heidegger's thoughts on Being to associate them with such philosophical baggage. For he mobilizes thinking Being not as a state, but as movement, and because of that seeks to destroy the ontotheological tradition that brings stasis to the process, to the event of Being that is Ereignis (Sheehan 1981). Indeed, as I seek to demonstrate in the reflections below on the Being of the body, awareness of its movement is precisely awareness of the body's Being as 'a processes of genesis and annihilation, of movement across thresholds and toward a limit.' When in *On Time and Being* (1972) Heidegger speaks of Ereignis as the 'ancient something,' he is referring not to an imperial, controlling past that will not go away, but, on the contrary, to the potential resistance that Being as movement has always posed for hypostatic, imperial, frameworks. Indeed, awareness of Ereignis packs tremendous powers of resistance precisely because it is an immediate insight into 'that process by which historical worlds and languages spring up, that happening which produces history, Being, world, and truth *as effects*' (Caputo 1986, xxiii).

Deleuze and Guattari (1987) posit desire as the flow of energy, the puissance, of human being/becoming/actuality, defining it as 'a process of production without reference to any exterior agency' (154). Desire is a power in and of itself, effectively prior to function, morality, or any other cultural reference. While desire is certainly operative in sexual reproduction, it is not confined either to reproduction or to genital sexuality. For Deleuze and Guattari, desire extends well beyond what is known generically as sex (love-making, casual genital encounters, sado-masochistic scenes, and the like). Desire is the force by which we move at all. *The movement of desire is the essence of the body.* As such, it is the process of all physical activities: walking, reading, writing, conversing, sitting, swimming, eating, defecating, thinking ... While Deleuze and Guattari ascribe tremendous importance to desire, they do not analyse its 'internal' dynamics. I suggest that reflection on the process of production will reveal not only how desire (puissance) is resourced by 'exterior agency' (pouvoir), but also the internal processual production of puissance that affords opportunities for resistance to pouvoir and may even offer freedom from such exterior agency.[12]

I think that one of the most striking potentials that emerges in aspects of the work of Deleuze and Guattari involves its resonance with elements of Buddhism. In such resonance lurks a powerful potential to break through the restrictive boundaries of traditional East–West dichotomies and exclusions, dichotomies that Said has identified in the racist projects of 'orientalism.' 'Orientalism,' Said (1978 [1994]) argues, differentiates East and West, thus producing a 'superior' West, which is fascinated by the 'exoticism' of the East but produces itself as pure by making the East decidedly other. (While Said is talking about the Middle East, the argument holds true for the Buddhist East as well.) This is true in many spheres, including the contemporary academic disciplines that for the most part perpetuate Western 'purity of thought.'[13] While it would require an entire book to build the case authoritatively, cultural studies, sociology, history, anthropology, psychology, and sport studies, as well as the ostensibly more radical intellectual trajectories of postmodernisms and queer theory, reproduce 'Western Identity' and 'Eastern Difference' through their exclusive engagement of 'Western' patterns of thought and exclusion of 'Eastern.' Given the exposure, indeed marketability, of 'Eastern' cultures, popularly in cuisine and to a lesser extent in music, it is remarkable that Euro-American academic discourse clings to the intellectual purity of 'Western' thought, producing a kind of intellectual xenophobia. These intellectual exclusions are as surely as anything territorializations of desire, of the intellectual desire to connect, to cross thresholds, which is the BwO.[14]

Robert Glass (1995) has made explicit connections between some postmodern writers (notably Martin Heidegger, Mark Taylor, Jacques Derrida, Emanuel Levinas, Thomas Altizer, and Deleuze and Guattari) and Zen Buddhism (specifically in the widely cited teachings of Dōgen Kigen) and explored some fascinating potentials for thinking across the borders of East and West through the complementary aspirations of Buddhism and postmodernism. The following invocation of elements of Eastern philosophies does not indicate my commitment to particular religious traditions, nor is it a synthesis of a vast array of spiritual traditions, which would be impossible. Rather, it is an exploration of alterity that is intended to open thinking about the body in ways that might transcend modern, Western, technological, and phallogocentric conceptions and practices of the body.

Emptiness

An essential dimension of Buddhist enlightenment is emptiness. Glass (1995) looks at two of the major interpretations of emptiness, which operate within a 'logic of negation': one considers it in the paradoxical emptiness of 'total presence,' and the other, in terms of abject difference. He suggests a 'third reading of emptiness,' which sees it in terms of 'affect, emotion, force, or desire' (1–2). Glass argues: 'Buddhist practice is best understood not as a matter of moving from thinking to non-thinking, but as a move from craving to compassion. Emptiness is not an achieved state of thinking (without thinking) but an achieved state of desire (compassion)' (3). There are similarities here with both Heidegger and Deleuze and Guattari. Heidegger aspired to a non-aggressive experience of reality that does not impose and produce reality according to the aggressive demands (which Buddhists call cravings) of human-centred projects, but instead is open to and cares for what lies beyond human-centred desire. Similarly, Deleuze and Guattari problematize the ways in which desire is socially, economically, and culturally produced to crave and therefore to realize itself according to the accumulative logics of capitalism. Instead, they envision a kind of desire that is open-ended. And a commitment to alterity suggests that desire can be open only when it comports itself compassionately with the potential for otherness and difference.

At the heart of Glass's project, and arguably of the several-thousand-year project of Buddhism(s), lies the practical pursuit of free modes of desire, of profoundly liberated ways of being, of becoming transcendent Bodies without Organs. A full exploration of the compatibility of Deleuze and Guattari with Buddhism is certainly beyond the scope of this book. Nevertheless, in the context of my eclectic use of texts, I would like to draw on Glass's 'third reading of emptiness' in Buddhism and postmodern thought in conjunction with Deleuze and Guattari, Heidegger, and others in order to develop a theory of the body that explores both its restrictive social construction and its liberating transcendental potential. Emptiness, I argue, is a compassionate and sacred gift that is the very source of the puissance of being free.

While Western eyes, particularly modern Western eyes, see Buddhism mostly as an esoteric religion with spiritual concerns that have little to do with the material problems of life, for its practitioners it is first and foremost a pragmatic approach to the problems of suffering. It employs a wide variety of meditative practices and rites (commensurate with the extensive range of historical Buddhist traditions) in order to clear away obstacles to happiness. That clearing comes preeminently from a practical and empirical appreciation of emptiness, which the Zen tradition calls *sunyata*. While there is a vast and varied Buddhist scholarly literature on emptiness as the ultimate nature of reality, generally the writers agree that the capacity to live happily with reality comes not from faith in religious teaching but from the empirical practice of embodying emptiness as a way of life.

Deleuze and Guattari also have an interest in the practical problems of embodying life free of abusive obstacles, be they the products of capitalism, sexism, humanism, or whatever. For them, this is a practical issue of deterritorializing the body, of entering into different ways of life that are not controlled by dominating and exploitive social constructions of embodied reality. As I pointed out above, Deleuze calls his 'philosophy' pragmatics – his is not an ideological framework to be embraced, but a practice of becoming different, which is liberatory. These practices, manifestations of desire, move in 'smooth space,' rather than in 'striated space.' Deleuze and Guattari say that it is the deterritorializing practice of desire that has an intensity of zero. Here is a powerful and practical resonance with Buddhist practice: emptiness is desire with an intensity of zero – i.e., without craving.

Emptiness, I now suggest, is essential to the freedom of movement that is the puissance of the body. The puissance of the living, desiring body is its production by movement. This process of production is the bodily play of presence and absence. Only in motion does the event of the body happen. Even when one is sitting still, the heart beats, the blood flows, the lungs expand and contract with air. What matters in the body's movement is not that it has gone from state A to state B (for example, lungs expanded to lungs contracted, or running from my house to the university); what matters is the eventfulness of the movement. Sometimes we are more aware of our movements than at other times; physical activities such as running, swimming, and sex can reveal an intensity in the event of the moving body that makes reflection more accessible. If I reflect, for instance, on running through one of my city's many beautiful ravines, I get the sense that being appears there as an event, an intense happening. Similarly in sitting meditation, following the movement of the breath, the puissance of movement can become astoundingly apparent.

An event happens. Being happens. Movement is implicit in the happening of an event; this is born out etymologically. Our English word 'event' comes from the Latin *eventus*, whose root is *venire*, which has its origins in the Greek root *BA*, which means 'go.' An event goes. This is not lost in modern English. For example: I might *go* for a run. Going for a run is not just a matter of preparing to run: getting dressed, warmed up, stretched, and ready to leave; actually moving through the course of my run, I am *going* running. Running is the way of this particular going. The event of my running consists of such a going. But this is not the sense of simply going away, of leaving behind. Going into that which lies before me is also coming. If I say that I am going into the ravine to run I am also coming into the ravine; these movements feel essentially the same. Coming, of course, is what the event of orgasm is often called (although it is now popularly spelled 'cumming'). Some people also call it 'going.'

'Going' and 'coming' refer to the same thing – the moving event of being. Reflecting on the event (*das Ereignis*) of the body's being, I draw the sense [*Sinn*] that the puissance of the body is active, not static. The eventful being of the body is its movement. The body *is* coming and going. A body that is not coming and going is an abstract body, devoid of being/becoming; it is not my body, the palpable body of my friend or lover; it is not the body that walks, runs, and swims. By moving, the body comes to presence, actualizes. Movement is the essence of the body. When the body completely ceases movement, it is no more. In death, after the flesh and organs have completed their decay and the bones have disintegrated, the movements of the body cease and the body as such is no more. In day-to-day speech, in medical and religious practices, we say that lack of movement marks the end of the life of the body; likewise, we say that movement's advent marks its inception. By moving, the body makes its reality. Movement is the primordial logos of the real for us who are embodied. Pigeons apparently cannot see unless they are moving – which is why they move their heads back and forth when they are walking. Similarly, we 'see' no reality without moving. If we are not moving, we are not. There is no reality for us without our own movements.

Understanding the body as movement is not just a philosophical clarification, a matter of refining the words that define the body. On the contrary, reflecting on the body as essentially moving, I suggest, undefines it, empties it of its distinction from everything else and allows its essential relatedness, its interdependence, with all elements of existence to show. Moving, we come and go in the sphere of essential openness, which is the puissance of the body.

In this meditation on the moving body, I go from a more or less familiar observation on the nature of movement experienced as presencing to thinking that goes beyond the logos of presence.

Movement appears in the play of presence and absence. In movement, absence is the opening, the clearing, the empty space, the freedom, through which presence is actualized. Absence opens presence, allows presence the freedom to be present. Absence is the essential 'space ahead' that allows presencing to happen, giving presence the very possibility of coming to presence. Absence draws presence into presence. Presence must have an absence into which it enters, or it will no longer be presencing.

Absence lies before presence, in anticipation. Just as absence lies in the foreground of presence, so too presence lies in the anticipation of absence. The absential anticipation of presence is the reception that absence gives presence. Absence must receive presence, or there will be no making present. In this anticipation of presence, absence draws presence. Thus drawn, presence penetrates absence.

The penetration of absence by presence need not be a violating assault on absence. Certainly in the phallogocentric cultures of patriarchal heterosexuality and its homosexual derivatives, penetration is an assault that establishes the power of penetrating males over submissive females or other males.[15] While this version of penetration may be the norm in phallocentric cultures, it need not be the gold standard. I admit that my use of the word 'penetration' does have genital sexual connotations that are especially sensitive in the context of oppressive power relations of gender in patriarchy. But my primary empirical point of reference is not genital sexuality. In fact my understanding of absence and presence, of the penetration of absence as an opening that makes presencing happen, comes from my athletic experience. It first occurred to me when I was lost in the intensity of working-out/playing on a rowing ergometer. I became aware of absence as the generous space that lay ahead of my exertions, drawing me into the wonderful opening that those exertions were. As my feet pressed against the stirrups and my upper body pulled the oar, my body both penetrated absence and was drawn into it.

Understanding penetration in the puissance of movement therefore requires purging it of its phallocentric associations. This is *not* the penetration of an 'inferior' other.[16] On the contrary, because it is the *essential* foreground of presence, absence is primordially *one* with presence. Being the foreground of presence, absence is essential to making present. Absence is the gift that makes presence possible. That is, in its gratuitous receptivity, absence opens presence in its own being-present; opening presence, absence draws presence into presence. Foregrounding presence, drawing presence into presence, absence inheres in presence.[17]

Because presence is the *event* of presencing (i.e., not a state but an occurrence), and because absence inheres in the event's happening, absence and presence are essentially one. As I run through the ravine near my house, my being there is both absence and presence, at once. I cannot be unless I am both absent and present, unless my presence and absence are fraught with one another. Heidegger speaks of this as *Ereignis*: the event of pres-absential *appropriation*, as it is usually translated (Sheehan 1983). But the word 'appropriation' is inadequate to the task, for it still echoes stasis and hierarchy in the sense of both the achievement of a state of appropriation and a pre-established appropriator. There is something simpler happening in movement, a primordial play that precedes any spirit of proprietorship. Absence draws presence into itself. Accordingly, drawing and penetrating are also one. Drawing-penetrating-absence-presence is the simple event of essential relatedness through which the body moves, by which the body is. It is a gift. Absence, here, is not therefore a lack; it is the inherent positive, productive, puissant generosity of moving. Absence is the gift that opens the event of our being/becoming. In its essence the event is complete. It is free. Indeed, the essence of freedom is this absence/presence play of movement.

Freedom

I began this reflection on the essence of the body with the observation that it is a moving event. That event, I suggested, is the puissant play of drawing-penetrating-absence-presence. What does the word 'play' suggest? 'Play' names activity. In sports we say that the ball is 'in play,' which means that it is engaged in the activity of playing ball. I play the violin, which means that together the violin and I produce music. 'Play' also connotes freedom, freedom for movement. The sail of a boat needs some play if it is to catch the wind. The play of the body is the freedom of presence and absence to draw and penetrate. This freedom is the *opening*, the absential, indeed *empty* space that actualizes the play of the body. The puissance of the body is its freedom to move. In 'On The Essence of Truth,' Heidegger (1961) says that the essence (the process of actualization) of truth is freedom, because freedom lets beings be the beings they are. The freedom of movement is the truth of the body. 'Movement,' 'play,' 'freedom,' 'truth' allude to some of the power (puissance) of the body. It is the power of the body to open.

'Open,' as I am using it here, is a gerund. This opening is not something static in the way that a door is an opening to a room. The opening of the body is a happening akin to the opening of flowers, a play, a dialogue, or a friendship. The body, I said above, is actualized through the opening that absence makes. Absence opens the space, as it were, for the body to *happen*; as such, absence is of the essence of the body, opening its reality. Absence is the clearing that makes possible the freedom of being/becoming. The true puissance of the body is thus the power of absence to actualize the freedom of movement in drawing-penetrating-absence-presence.

What kind of desire, what 'process of production' (Deleuze and Guattari 1987, 154), realizes this puissant freedom of the body? Above, I quoted Massumi (1992): '*Puissance* refers to a range of potential. Deleuze has defined it as a "capacity for existence," "a capacity to affect or be affected" [which refers not to emotion, but to the augmentation or diminution of the body's capacity to act], a capacity to multiply connections' (Massumi 1992, xvii). How is this capacity realized in a way that is true, that opens the body in its freedom? Recall that the philosophy of the limit obliges us to be open to that which lies outside any system by virtue of its being a system; this is the commitment to alterity. Desire that seeks realization in alterity needs to be free of systematizing blinkers. In order to be free, it needs to be a kind of desire that does not project (Heidegger's *ta mathemata*) onto the body a framework for understanding, thus producing a reality that being known in advance prestructures the shape of (perceived) reality.

In *The Experience of Freedom*, Jean-Luc Nancy (1993) works through the question of freedom in the work of Kant, Adorno, and Heidegger and argues that freedom cannot be grounded in any system of thought, but must instead be experienced: 'An experience is first of all an encounter with any given, or rather, in a less simply positive vocabulary, it is the testing of something real (in any case, it is the act of a thought which does not conceive, or interrogate, or construct what it thinks except by being already taken up and cast as thought by its thought). Also, according to the origin of the word "experience" in *peir_* and in *ex-periri*, an experience is an attempt executed without reserve, given over to the *peril* of its own lack of foundation and security in this "object" of which it is not the subject but [is] instead the passion, exposed like the pirate (*peir_t_s*) who freely tries his luck on the high seas. In a sense, which here might be the first and last sense, freedom, to the extent that it is the thing itself of thinking, cannot be appropriated, but only "pirated": its "seizure" will always be illegitimate' (20).

Nancy's is a decidedly empirical freedom, with a standard for empiricism that is far more rigorous than that of the so-called empirical sciences that I criticized above in chapter 1. Nancy suggests that freedom must be an experience of alterity, in which we do not cling to the grounding of our various concepts, including the concept of Self, but where instead we remain open to the potential of being completely altered, even perhaps undone, by the encounter. This is alterity – openness to being altered.

The truly empirical encounter with freedom therefore does not secure a ground for the freedom-seeking subject. Indeed, 'the inability of the subject to procure a ground on which it can support itself does not require further work or deeper labour; it demands the abandonment of the idea of subjectivity in favor of the thought of abandonment, of existence, of freedom' (Nancy 1993, xxiv). Here, suggests Nancy, is 'a free beginning for thought. "Thinking" would no longer mean making indissoluble distinctions and seeking solid grounds; thinking would be exposure to dissolution and groundlessness' (xxii). Such thinking therefore needs to be free of the gravity of the grounded systems of thought of the disciplines – physics, biology, physiology, psychology, sociology, history, philosophy, even language itself ... Grounded in systematic thinking, we are subject to the force of gravity that the parergonality of the system exerts on the possibilities of experience. Where grounded, we are subject to the gravity of the ground. The root of the word 'gravity' is 'grave.' The desire that would realize the freedom and therefore the truth of the body should not be desire that pulls us into the grave that systems dig for us. This desire needs an anti-gravitational force.

The desire that engages the freedom of puissance needs to be a production of desire that is not a subject-presence (Self as *hupokeimenon*) making demands on absence, grasping at absence to ground the future in some re-production of the present. It should not marshal absence as a resource for the aggressive reproduction of presence, making absence obey the projections of the self-presencing self. It needs to be a production of desire that exists by virtue of its openness to the radically altering potential of absence. For those of us who experience life by an attachment to reality as it appears in our presence, who routinely go about our lives by projecting our present selves into the future, in order to shape absence in a way that conforms to some pre-established trajectory that we seem to be following, being truly open to the potential of absence is probably terrifying. Indeed, for the ground-craving (gravitational) subject, the complete openness of absence that constitutes movement seems far from the wonderful, gratuitous gift to which I have alluded in the past few pages. As Nancy points out, experience is perilous. From the perspective of the self-grounding subject, the experience of absence is the abject gap, the abyss that must be avoided at all costs (Taylor 1987). And the greatest cost of all, the cost that most of us are all too willing to pay, is the cost of giving up the true freedom of the body. We pay dearly for the 'comfort' of our abjection, as I show in the next chapter. But our willingness to purchase our holiday from the abyss is not just a personal flaw of weak individuals. It is, in a more sinister vein, one of the complex exploitive strategies of pouvoir, which I get to below.

The freedom of presence-becoming-absence therefore is not just an easy ride in the ecstatic abyss of joyful abandon. Indeed, the philosophy of clearing and openness, as Glass trenchantly observes, opens the grievous danger of clearing the way for evil. Not just moral depravity, but what Immanuel Kant calls 'absolute evil' (1965, 87–8n), which Hannah Arendt in *The Origins of Totalitarianism* (1968) rephrases as 'radical evil,' looms in our potential for freedom. In Nancy's philosophy, terrible possibilities burden the experience of freedom. For Nancy, this must be the case for freedom to be truly free. Arguably, murders, rapists, and torturers – not to mention exploitive and environmentally destructive global capital markets and their consumers – experiment with freedom. Freedom that trades in abuse, however, is not ultimately free, because then the free experience of one person, or social group, depends on the restriction of another. From a holistic perspective, that is only partial freedom. Such 'freedom' is only the misperception of freedom from the partial and selfish perspective of the abuser. Obviously, it is not the freedom of alterity. The radical experience of freedom and therefore truth must transcend the confines of the self that produces its freedom by subtracting the same from others. Glass's 'Third Reading of Emptiness in Buddhism and Postmodern Thought' (in Glass 1995) offers the potential to foster desire that is radically free precisely by its ethical commitment to the alteritous task of guarding the freedom of the 'other,' from the pseudo-freedom of self-ish others.

The experience of freedom in the puissance of the body emerges, I suggest, in an enlightened engagement with absence. To explore this claim, I first review Glass's first, second, and third readings of emptiness as approaches to 'enlightened engagement.' I then apply the third as an alteritous approach to the drawing-penetrating-absence-presence event of movement (Ereignis) that allows ethical freedom and therefore truth to happen in that which is most near to us: movement.[18] This requires reflective thinking, which means, as Heidegger has said, 'to dwell on what lies close and meditate on what is closest; upon that which concerns us, each one of us, here and now; *here*, on this patch of home ground; *now* in the present hour of history' (1966a, 47).

Glass says that the Buddhist understanding of emptiness (*sunyata*) is frequently identified with mental processes, in which the goal of meditation practice is to move from thinking to pure non-thinking and in this way to become less attached and therefore more attuned to and accepting of the impermanence of life. This occurs in the practice of meditation (*zazen*), in which the profound simultaneous presencing of everything appears in their interrelatedness: 'There is a shift from attachment to non-attachment through a specific practice of thinking understood here as the "presencing" of all that is. Externally, this "presencing" results in an understanding of the "interrelationality" of all things' (Glass 1995, 32). Here the practice of meditation itself is enlightenment, an ultimate emptying of attachment to the world. Glass draws parallels between this 'first' Buddhist reading of emptiness and Heidegger's similar concept of *Gelassenheit* – i.e., the individual's release from the aggressive, calculative, domineering thinking that characterizes the history of Western thought and culminates in the nihilism of the modern technological project. In this reading of emptiness, both sunyata and Gelassenheit are processes of 'letting be' – it is the emptiness of non-interference that arises from a profound insight into oneness, the letting be of the fulness of presence.

Glass is critical of this reading of emptiness, saying that its neutrality makes it ethically inadequate. Pure acceptance and letting be let all manner of things be, both good and evil. Certainly from the ethical perspective of the philosophy of the limit, it does not engage in alteritous guardianship. As Cornell (1992) observes: 'The entire project of the philosophy of the limit is driven by the ethical desire to enact the ethical relation ... the aspiration to a nonviolent relationship to the Other and to otherness more generally, that assumes responsibility to guard the Other' (2). Glass argues that while the first reading is nonviolent in its letting-be, its lack of necessary engagement means that it falls significantly short of being an ethic of care.

Glass's second (and also critical) reading of emptiness comes from the deconstructionist work of Mark Taylor, especially as he is influenced by Derrida's work on *différence*, which Glass (1995) identifies as 'an irreparable tear': 'In Heidegger that which guides decision-making is the wish to maintain a poetic mode of presencing, while in Taylor it is the recognition of the edge/rift/tear/difference which must not (or rather cannot) ever be suppressed ... There is a play between word and nothing, silence and speech, light and dark with neither one dominant. Emptiness is now an interdependent opposite of fullness with both playing back and forth as equal partners' (38, 41).

From this perspective, presence is derivative of *différence*. Emptiness in this reading allows to remain open the open space, the gap, the wound that is our condition and that can never be articulated, for which there is no soothing antidote. In this particularly postmodern reading, emptiness means leaving this gap alone, not trying to tie it together into a tidy (Hegelian-like) unity. Glass criticizes this reading in a similar vein to that of the first: it is a mental exercise of learning to accept a reality non-violently – in this case, the violence would be the attempt to close the wound of difference. Highlighting the ethical, Glass (1995) says: 'Accepting the work of difference in the process of thinking does not compel one to respect difference in relating to others. Or, to reverse the point, the internal working of difference is not dependent on any particular external action' (58). While the laudable imperative of this reading of emptiness is non-violence in the face of difference, it holds the fact of difference and the ethics of difference to be independent of actual ethical action. The truth of difference is unrelated to possible practical engagements with it. Emptiness here is only an intellectual enterprise, not an ethics of engaged care, which, Glass argues, his third reading of emptiness, offers.

The third reading of emptiness is, I think, particularly helpful for my project here. Its emphasis on the *practice* of desire serves the pragmatic venture that underlies this book: how do we free the body with an ethics of alterity? How do we become open to the truth of the body? This reading of emptiness emerges out of the Buddhist insight that the self/ego is a problematic construction that is perpetuated by grasping, craving self-interest. The self-grounding self fails to see and produce reality in a way that engages and cares for the profound interdependence that is the essence of all life on earth, indeed of the being of the entire universe. Glass explains this engagement by reference to traditional Buddhist concepts of interdependence, with which he also makes analogies to quantum physics. The project of the third reading of emptiness is to be able to see beyond the self and to live in a way that transcends selfishness. I expand this below and suggest that such emptying allows enlightened desire to transcend the various social constructions of being human.

From traditional Buddhism, Glass calls on the complementary myths of 'Indra's Net' and 'One Bright Pearl.' He sites Francis Cook's description of the myth of Indra's Net: 'Far away in the heavenly abode of the great god Indra, there is a wonderful net that has been hung ... in such a manner that it stretches out infinitely in all directions ... A single glittering jewel hangs in each "eye" of the net, and since the net itself is infinite in all dimensions, the jewels are infinite in number ... If we now arbitrarily select one of the jewels for inspection, and look closely at it, we will discover that in its polished surface there are reflected all other jewels in the net, infinite in number. Not only that, but each of the jewels reflected in this one jewel is also reflecting all the other jewels, so that there is an infinite reflecting process occurring' (Cook 1977, 2). 'Each jewel is thus positioned to reflect and be reflected in all the others. When one is able to practice non-attachment, one then authenticates one's original nature reflecting and being reflected in all other jewels' (Glass 1995, 32).

Non-attachment here means not to be grounded in one's self-construction. This, I suggest, involves an openness to absence that does not project the present and socially constructed self into absence out of a (neurotic and habitual) attachment to presence. Non-attachment allows the self to reflect the infinity of reflecting jewels. So rather than projecting itself onto others, this desire reflects the others. It shares the infinite passion (compassion) of the infinity of reflecting jewels rather than imposing the passion of the finite self onto an otherwise-infinite reality. Freed of our attachments to our self-projections onto the real, we can appreciate and live in an infinitely reflective interdependent reality. When applied to my analysis of movement, Indra's net suggests that being open to the space of absence, which is that which is closest to us, allows a reflective capacity to emerge, a mirror that shows how we are inextricably entwined with everything. The practice of emptiness clears the debris that obfuscates the interdependence of reality. 'The clarity of this mirror reflects and is reflected in other mirrors. Therefore, whatever appears in one's own mirror-self is contingent upon the state of other mirror selves. Any one "self" is inextricably bound up with all other "selves." There can be no separate selves when each individual self is at least partly constructed in relationship with others' (Glass 1995, 74).

This is a profoundly ecological approach to understanding and making reality. The myth of Indra's Net and the notion of the infinite interconnectedness of reality being reflected in each jewel – that is, in each particularity, both human and otherwise – constitute another way of expressing the transpersonal dimension that Levin insists is part of the phenomenon of the body. Teilhard de Chardin (1959) also believed that the issue here is not an individual matter, arguing that improvement in our condition is a profoundly interdependent matter: 'The outcome of the world, the gates of the future, the entry into the super-human – these are not thrown open to a few of the privileged nor to one chosen people to the exclusion of all others. They will open only to an advance of all together.' Similarly the transpersonal has analogies with Merleau-Ponty's (1968) idea of the pre-personal field of the flesh, the intertwining, the chiasm. It also shares something with Deleuze and Guattari's BwO, the unrestrained power of connection that is the body's potential in the infinity of reflecting jewels. For Deleuze and Guattari, however, processes of territorialization and reterritorialization rein in that power – an issue I discuss when I speak below of pouvoir.

The point here is that the phenomenon of movement can realize the reflectivity of the body's infinite potential and interconnectedness. Emptiness allows that infinity to be actualized, to be reality. In the drawing-penetrating-absence-presence dynamics of movement, emptiness is a kind of desire that does not project into absence the grounded self, but instead can transcend the self. This transcendence is expressed in the experience of a kind of ultimately unified reality that does not obliterate difference. Dōgen expresses this in the enigmatic concept of One Bright Pearl. 'The entire universe is one bright pearl' (Glass 1995, 75).

Glass explains his third reading of this emptiness by drawing an analogy with the wave-particle theory of light: 'Dōgen states: "We do not speak of two or three pearls, and so the entirety is one True Dharma Eye, the *Body* of Reality, One Expression. The entirety is brilliant light, One Mind"' (Cook 1977, 74, emphasis added).

> If 'the entirety is brilliant light' is a description of Dōgen's emptiness, and light has both a particle and wave nature, then seeing emptiness as having two natures may be helpful in understanding its behaviour. Perhaps Indra's Net is better visualized not only as a net of interconnected particle-selves but also as a wave of brilliant light. This wave of light is not static but moves, and exerts a 'force' upon the particle-selves. The net as a whole then takes on the characteristics of the force of the larger wave. Wave, then, embraces particle, but particle does not embrace wave. Seeing the net as light does not negate its particle nature, nor does seeing the light as a set of interconnected particles negate its wave nature – once the action of the wave upon particle is realized. Following this analogue through to the end, the goal of practice [of enlightened desire] would then be to dwell upon one's 'particle-nature' while realizing 'wave-nature' is primary and governs behaviour. This requires not only a shift in focus from particle to wave but a shift in the mode of awareness that guides action, from particle sensitivities to wave sensitivities.' (Glass 1995, 78)

This practice of emptiness produces desire through selves that manifest primarily the whole rather than desire that manifests primarily the particular. Emphasis becomes the discerning point of desire. Glass's third reading of emptiness opens the possibility of particular selves, which I have called grounded self-presencing selfhood, with the capacity to experience and indeed to create reality that significantly and ultimately transcends that grasping particularity. In the context of movement, emptiness would be desire that is produced in the self, and is highly aware of the self, but does not insist on making the self the foundation for the opening of absence. Emptiness here is the creative discerning power to realize the movement of the body in the brilliant wave of light, to actualize, in the dynamics of drawing-penetrating-absence-presence, not the primacy of the particular socially constructed self, but the primacy of the Body of Reality, which is the wave of the entire universe that the 'singular glittering jewel' of the particular body reflects.

This enlightened realization of the nature of the entire universe is not 'knowledge' of the entire universe, as though one were a god. Nor is it knowledge of the sort that Stephen Hawking and other astrophysicists seek in a grand unified theory. It is not a *concept* of the entire universe. The enlightenment of emptiness does not attempt to contain reality by arriving at the ultimate intellectual representation of it in its fundamental principles. It is much simpler than that. The enlightenment of the third reading of emptiness is desire. It is a desiring production of reality in the movement of the body that is open to absence. Rather than moving into absence with the fear and loathing of abjection, emptiness is drawn to absence compassionately. It is openness without limits. Emptiness is full alterity. This compassionate desire is pure, unfettered love. In such love there is no abyss, no abjection, no fear, no loathing. Instead there is a profound acceptance.

The gift of absence is produced compassionately, in the love of the impermanence of movement, rather than in the fear of it. Rather than fearfully grasping at some static ground (grave-ity), emptiness as compassionate desire loves the impermanence of the body. The love of impermanence is the Body of Reality about which Dōgen speaks; it is the transcendent desire that flows with the wave of impermanence, which is the way of the entire universe, which makes it One Bright Pearl. Every event of Ereignis is a jewel that reflects that One Bright Pearl, in the flow of movement. Glass (1995) concludes: 'Buddhist practice is best presented not as a move from one form of thinking to another (from thinking to without thinking) but as a move from one nature of desire to another (from craving to compassion). What distinguishes the third reading from the first two is that Buddhist practice is not seen as an achieved state of thinking but as an achieved state of desire' (83).

Embodying Emptiness

Compassionate desire as a practice rather than as the disengaged acceptance of the thought of emptiness (the first and second readings) is necessary for the freedom and truth that I am suggesting is a potential path of desire in the production of movement that is the essence of the body's puissance. For the drawing-penetrating-absencing-presencing that is the event (Ereignis) of the body is not just a thought, a philosophical disposition, or a mental state that needs to be acknowledged in its truth. The event of the body is precisely an engagement with the production of drawing-penetrating-absence-presence. In other words, the kind of desire that occurs there makes a significant difference to the reality that is produced. Desire is productive.

Enlightened engagement with, indeed the production of, reality is not just an acknowledgment of a state of affairs. From the perspective that Glass and I are suggesting, enlightenment is a form of desire that produces compassionate reality. Emptiness is therefore a practice that produces an empty reality, and the production of that reality forms the practice of emptiness. It has the form of an emptying hermeneutic circle. Emptiness has the meaning of an entirely alteritous gift. It imposes no meaning on the space of absence; it simply gives it the freedom to be what it is: smooth, free space. 'Emptiness' then is not a representation of reality, but a word that points to an embodied practice of openness, of embodied alterity. Thus to understand 'emptiness,' one needs to leave it outside the parergonality of the representative thinking that characterizes dominant Western modes of understanding and enter into its flow as a production of desire. Emptiness is therefore a sacred practice of opening that cannot in its truth be named but can only be entered, without the projections of language.

Enlightened movement – the body of enlightenment, the body of ultimate reality – is the practice of movement that is produced in compassionate, non-aggressive desire. In this movement of the body, the relations of presence and absence are compassionate, rather than aggressive. Presence does not press itself on absence, forcing absence to reproduce presence, which is narcissistic movement. Similarly absence is not an abject threat to the event of presence. It is instead the freedom that allows presence to become different, altered, to move beyond the confines of its pre-construction. Crucial to this is the lack of fear. Enlightened desire, the 'Body of Reality,' is fearless. This is a practice of desire that produces an empty space for movement. As I argued above from Heidegger, the essence of truth is freedom, which means that the most truthful space for the movement of the body is a free space. Deleuze is very interested in this space, for that free space is the body that is free, desire that is free. He characterizes this freedom as 'smooth space.' Smooth space does not constrain the freedom of movement. Rather than demanding that movement be produced in accordance with some discourse (which Deleuze calls striated space – movement is forced along prepossessed discursive lines), smooth space is open. Empty desire allows that openness to happen and in so doing produces reality that is free.

The production of this smooth space, the realization of enlightened movement, the practice of free desire is both extraordinarily simple and difficult to realize. The simple part is that absence, the pres-absentiality of movement (in drawing-penetrating-absence-presence), being essentially empty, is free. And whether you want it or not, it awaits you. Not just some time in the future, but right now. Or as Deleuze and Guattari (1987) answer the question of how to make yourself a BwO, 'You have one (or several). It's not so much that it pre-exists or is ready-made, although in certain respects it is pre-exis-tent ... You can't desire without making one' (149). It is, in other words, inevitable. The complex part is that that freedom is seldom given pri-macy. Indeed it is very far from modern, capitalist, technological, phallologocentric productions of reality. I turn below to that produc-tion of reality under the name 'pouvoir' and consider it in relation to the enlightened freedom of desire that I am addressing here.

Where the freedom/truth of the body does not receive primacy, the work of emptiness is compassionately to empty reality of the aggres-sive insistence of those discourses that re-source the puissant power of the body's movement. This can be done only holistically, with the primacy of the wave of light as the inspiration for and texture of movement. If we keep in mind the myths of Indra's Net and One Bright Pearl and the essential interconnectedness of reality, then it is clear that this is something that individuals alone cannot accomplish. Each individual (particle) is a reflection of the infinite whole (one bright pearl). So if the whole (wave) of desire is not moving in smooth space, then no particle is either.

Appreciating our essential connectedness in the wave is important. Deleuze and Guattari refer to it as *the* BwO. But I think that it can be more meaningful to us if we call it instead *our* BwO. Individuals stand out from their profoundly shared Body of Reality. *The* BwO stresses BwO as somehow removed from our immediacy. Whereas *our* BwO suggests that we are all in this together.

We can realize the Buddhist holistic understanding of the essential connectedness or interdependence of all that is, I suggest, from a Deleuzian perspective in the power of the body that I have referred to as puissance. Reiterating Massumi (1992): '*Puissance* refers to a range of potential. It has been defined by Deleuze as a "capacity for existence," "a capacity to affect or be affected," a capacity to multiply connections' (xvii). The body's potential to affect, to be affected, and to multiply connections can be realized in the body's connective power, visualized as a reflective jewel in Indra's Net. Here the multiplicity of connections is infinite. The infinite connections of this myth suggest the opposite of the desire that T.S. Eliot spoke of when he described hell in Dante's Inferno as 'where nothing connects with nothing' (Kumar 2000). We could say that this is 'heavenly' desire, where everything connects with everything.

Deleuze and Guattari mobilize a number of metaphors in order to open the imaginative potentials of desire in this respect. Among them are the contrasting metaphors of arborescence and rhizomatics. The arborescent model of desire understands it as highly organized and restricted according to function, all of which is centralized in a great unbending trunk – the oak tree, the great immovable symbolic tree of Western phallologocentric knowledge, is the authoritative archetype of this way of life and desire for stasis, order, and security. In contrast to this, Deleuze and Guattari (1987) imagine the metaphor of the rhizome: 'In contrast to centred (even polycentric) systems with hierarchical modes of communication and preestablished paths, the rhizome is an acentered, nonhierarchical, nonsignifying system without a General and without an organizing memory or central automaton, defined solely by a circulation of states. What is at question in the rhizome is a relation to sexuality – but also to the animal, the vegetal, the world, politics, the book, things natural and artificial – that is totally different from the arborescent relation: all manners of "becomings"' (21).

This is desire that opens freely. It is not restricted to the parergonal logics of systems, centres, hierarchies, signs. It is the desire of alterity, the desire that is free to be altered by the productive opening of absence, free to become different from the desire reproduced in the established work of cultures, species, kinds. Just as Indra's Net has no governing centre, hierarchy, or semiotic structure, but an infinity of multiplying connections, so too the diffusion of the rhizome sends it beyond structural controls. Two similar metaphors for alteritous desire, emanating out of two very different historical traditions – Indra's net and the rhizome.

One way to think of the net and the rhizome is to think of them as idealized static structures that may or may not be reproduced in the practices of life. As such they are metaphors for an ideal existence to which we might aspire. But such understanding, by reifying the metaphorical structure, lacks the truly radical transformative power of eventfulness (*Ereignis*) that I am suggesting is the power of puissance. Moreover, it suggests an economy of desire that is organized around, indeed governed by, a quest for the resolution of the difference between lived reality and a philosophical metaphor for reality. That is a teleological economy in which the expenditure of desire is directed at the achievement of a resolution. It participates in aspects of the problematic historical construction to which Glass refers in his second reading of emptiness viz the work of Mark Taylor.

In *Altarity*, Taylor (1987) suggests that one of modernity's hallmarks is the desire to erase difference. Philosophically this desire is epitomized in Hegel's master synthesis in the Absolute Knowledge of his System. Similarly, it shows in the long-standing Western phallologocentric will to power that seeks control over all that is different from Western thought and projects. Its antecedents extend to the Christology of Jesus of Nazareth, by which the church attempted to overcome the difference between God and man, through the myth of the unifying sacrifice of Jesus, the Christian man-God. Most important, this way of thinking and desiring constructs desire in the logic of a lack that can be fulfilled, which then traps the freedom of desire in the parergonal logic of teleological fulfilment.

> In contrast to these approaches is Deleuze's strategy of plateaux, taken from Gregory Bateson. 'A plateau is always in the middle, not at the beginning or end ... Gregory Bateson uses the word "plateau" to designate something very special: a continuous, self-vibrating region of intensities whose development avoids any orientation toward a climax or external end ... It is a regrettable characteristic of the Western mind to relate expressions and actions to exterior or transcendent ends, instead of evaluating them on a plane of consistency on the basis of their extrinsic value ... We call a "plateau" any multiplicity connected to other multiplicities by superficial underground stems in such a way as to form or extend a rhizome' (Deleuze and Guattari 1987, 21–2). 'Every BwO is itself a plateau in communication with other plateaus on the plane of consistency.' (158)

This invocation of 'plateau,' I suggest, deepens an appreciation of the energy suggested in the metaphor of Indra's Net. That infinite net, which is infinite in *all* directions, is not a metaphorical object of stasis, but is rather a 'continuous, self-vibrating region of intensities whose development avoids any orientation towards a climax or external end.' An empirical encounter with the reality to which this metaphor alludes suggests, at least in my experience, that the inter-reflectivity of the infinite jewels is there precisely in the vibrations produced in the paradox of their *mutual* reality. As Deleuze and Guattari (1987) point out, it is a matter of experiencing reality from the midst of the event, of being immersed *in* the event. This is the decidedly non-Western perspective of being without ground, of seeing neither from the top nor from the bottom, neither from before nor from after, but from within the midst. And on the plateau, in the midst of the vibration of the real, there is no beginning or end, no difference of kinds: 'Never is a plateau separable from the cows that populate it, which are also the clouds in the sky' (23). 'A rhizome has no beginning or end; it is always in the middle, between things, *intermezzo*. The tree is filiation, but the rhizome is alliance, uniquely alliance. The tree imposes the verb "to be," but the fabric of the rhizome is the conjunction, "and ... and ... and ..." This conjunction carries enough force to shake and uproot the verb "to be." Where are you going? Where are you coming from? What are you heading for? These are totally useless questions. Making a clean slate, starting or beginning again from ground zero, seeking a beginning or a foundation – all imply a false conception of voyage, and *movement*' (25, emphasis added).

It is through the groundlessness of the plateau, the unutterable gratuity of the event of Ereignis, that the essential freedom of the moving body, that the infinite reflections and vibrations of Indra's Net, that the Body of Reality, becomes manifest. In Dōgen's metaphor of One Bright Pearl, rhizomatics apply by appreciating that the 'body of reality' moves from the middle. (It is no coincidence that many Eastern arts such as tai chi, chi kung, and ikido locate the point of the body's energy in the middle of the body, a few inches below the navel on most people. In tai chi this place is called *tan t'ien*. In Zen practice it is the *hara*, and it is the opening to infinity. This is the pearl in the middle of an individual body that is actually the reflection of all the other pearls in the universe – it is understood to be immensely powerful.) 'Proceeding from the middle, coming and going, rather than starting and finishing ... The middle is by no means an average; on the contrary, it is where things pick up speed. *Between* things does not recognize a localizable relation going from one thing to the other and back again, but a perpendicular direction, a transversal movement that sweeps one *and* the other away, a stream without beginning or end that undermines its banks and picks up speed in the middle' (Deleuze and Guattari 1987, 25).

Applied to my reflections on movement, the rhizomatic production of reality does not produce the real by projecting presence into an absence that has been programmed to be a particular future drawn out of the organizing and grounding principles of the past. Instead, the rhizome, vibrating in the middle of the plateau, remains open to the perpendicular alteritous potential that is manifest when desire does not try to reproduce itself on the horizontal plane of linear space–time. Annie Dillard calls this perpendicular temporal direction 'vertical eternity' (Dillard 1982).

The plateau can become more apparent in the intense experience of movement. I have found it to be particularly the case in running, swimming, cycling, dancing, as well as sitting meditation, and, occasionally, sex. Certainly when I am in the middle of these things, when I am aware of the plateau, 'things pick up speed,' and the speed is not confined to the horizontal, linear spatio-temporal plane. On the plateau, drawing-penetrating-absence-presence is freed, opening into every plane, every dimension of Indra's Net.

The puissance of the moving body, of its being, is the freedom that allows rhizomatic becoming. Such becoming, which is the puissant self-penetration of the body event of drawing-penetrating-absence-presence, is limitless. This is the limitlessness of inwardlyness: penetrating itself, presence presses inwardly into itself. *Self-penetrating, inwarding movement can have no limits.* Limitless inwarding movement is the coming and going of being, the 'direction' of self-penetration. The meaning of inward here is crucial. This is *not* inward in the sense of going into the Self, of focusing on oneself. This is inward in the sense of going into the wholeness of becoming. The 'in' of 'inward' here connotes the sense of the word 'in,' as when we speak of being in tune, in harmony, or in love. Inward is the direction of eternity.

Heraclitus, whose fragments Heidegger argues echo a reality that has been lost in the West since the dawn of the Greek classical age, observes: 'It is wise to agree that all things are one.' One Bright Pearl shines in the reflective luminosity of the middle, the plateau of desire that is manifest in the event of the moving body – at least in those productions of desire that do not grasp at absence trying to secure the particularity of a historical past, present, and future. Deleuze and Guattari speak of something similar, calling it our non-limitive BwO, which is not a thing, but an ongoing, eventful dimension of energy. Merleau-Ponty alludes to this essential relatedness as the body's prepersonal communicative power. Levin (1985), pointing to the importance of our bodily motility, draws together Heidegger's thoughts on being-as-a-whole and Merleau-Ponty's on the prepersonal dimension of the body, saying that through our motility and thus our 'primordial attunement by Being as a whole, what we encounter, along the way, is a *prepersonal* and, in fact a *transpersonal* dimension' (97). For Merleau-Ponty (1968), that transpersonal dimension is the intertwining, the chiasm by which we are immersed in the life of the flesh, a fleshiness that is crucially beyond the merely individual configuration of flesh that we associate with individual people. He says that our carnality is the way in which we are present in a vast, intertwining, fleshly reality, which we have in common with all carnal life. That chiasm, moreover, is a source of meaning that is more 'ancient than thought' and freer than discourse. I suggest that by moving in emptiness, and by paying attention to moving, we can learn the meaning of our immersion in the flesh and thus apprehend the meanings of being/becoming as more than a subjective, personal, self-grounded experience.

So the essence of the body as puissance is its coming to presence by moving (drawing-penetrating-absence-presence), which is itself essentially playful, free, limitless, productive desire, which is the power of our essential relatedness to everything. This, I have argued, is realized in the practice of emptiness. Contrary to disembodied conceptual approaches to emptiness, which Glass critiqued in his first two readings, the practice of emptiness is a profoundly embodied practice. I would add that, as such, it is an erotic practice. I spoke above of logos and defined it as an openness to being that gathers together and lays before us what is there in the form of a hermeneutic circle, which allows it to appear in the analogies of meaning structures (Heidegger 1975). And I said that there are different logoi, such as technology and gender.

There is also a logos that gathers together the essence of the body as puissance. The Greeks understood this logos in the myth of the god Eros. Our erotic capacity is an openness to being that gathers together and lays before us the puissance of our essential relatedness to all elements of becoming such that the relationship is meaningful, not simply a concept, as in the various metaphors that I have invoked from Buddhism and Deleuze and Guattari.[19] Eros is the mythical god of connection, the god of movement, the god of the body becoming our BwO. In other words, Eros opens the meaning of the puissance of our carnality, of our moving being, our eventful impermanence, which is the ultimate Body of Reality.

Eros can bring us to the empty space in which alterity can happen. This is why Eros is so feared, and why it has been so thoroughly policed, disciplined, and punished by regimes that prefer closure to openness. Deleuze and Guattari speak of Eros as the 'energy dedicated to the connective syntheses [the middle] at the basis of becoming' (Massumi 1992, 192 n43). Eros manifests the body's potential for infinite freedom as well as its contrary availability as a resource for technology. The extent and quality of our appreciation of Eros therefore can have a profound effect on how we go about life. Where it is compassionately empty, Eros manifests freedom. Where Eros is discursively loaded, tyranny lurks.

Empty desire, which is a profound, compassionate erotic openness to the freedom of movement, seems very far from the desire that is so familiar to those of us who live in the worlds of modern capitalist technology. For many readers, the discussion above may have referred to a phenomenon so removed from their reality that it has been incomprehensible. Buddhist practice appreciates that incomprehensibility and makes the realization of emptiness in the face of its seeming impossibility the focus of its work. I now attempt to explain the possible incomprehensibility of empty desire by exploring the ways in which the modern technological project configures and resources the puissance of the body. My argument is that that project has been so successful that it is difficult to imagine any other reality. The form of desire that embodies that project is pouvoir.

But before moving on, I would like to reiterate that I do not intend my invocation of the above myths and metaphors to suggest any ontological priority for their structures. For there are many, many ways of alluding to the potential manners of becoming to which these point. Surely this is the multifaceted history of the ways in which cultures have dealt with the 'sacred.' I have focused particularly on Buddhism and on Deleuze and Guattari, not so as to restrict reflection to a long-standing philosophical tradition (Buddhism) and a contemporary psycho-political program (Deleuze and Guattari), but in a modest attempt to open the range for thinking about the body and the potential for truthful, liberating ways of being/becoming. My aim has been, as David Farrell Krell (1997) concludes in the introduction to *Archeticture* [sic] *Ecstasies of Space, Time and the Human Body*, 'a matter of breaking up frames of reference, or of rejoining ancient yet still unfamiliar frames of reference, allowing an ecstatic space for something *other* to approach us' (8).

Pouvoir

Classical sociology (Weber), psychoanalysis (Freud), and critical theory (Marcuse) analysed the problem of desire in modernity as a problem of repression, which Foucault has called the 'repressive hypothesis.' Weber, believing that there was a close relationship between the rise of industrial capitalism and Protestant asceticism, said that the Protestant sense of 'calling,' self-denial, and hard work served a social function in the 'rational ordering of the body which was thus protected from the disruptions of desire in the interests of continuous factory production' (Turner 1984, 100). Freud's psychodynamics posits the 'primal repression' of libido, which blocks and prevents primitive, forbidden impulses of the id from entering consciousness, thus controlling the potential for wild, libidinous behaviour. Marcuse (1969) suggests that the capitalist system, in order to produce surplus capital, maximizes production by minimizing social resistance in the form of libidinous power by systematically repressing sexual desire; this results in concomitant surplus repression.

Following Heidegger, Foucault, and Deleuze and Guattari, I suggest that the modern body/desire is not *repressed* in the service of social forces, but is rather *developed* for its potential as a resource. From Heidegger, I speak of the aggressive marshalling of being, which he calls *Gestell*, as a way of dealing with the body as puissance that radically transforms the body in the production of resources. To explain that transformation, I call on Foucault's concept of the subjection of the body under the 'governing' powers of knowledge, discipline, and biopolitics. From Deleuze and Guattari, I speak of the coding and decoding of the flows of desire that territorialize and deterritorialize the body as processes of limiting or freeing the body. I bring together these three theories in this definition of pouvoir: the aggressive resourcing/wasting of puissance by processes of coding and discipline.

As we saw above, the essence of modern technology is the aggressive disposition of humans and other beings as resources and waste according to their use-value. The danger here is that technology reveals our being according to projects that are not sensitive to the essential freedom and truth of our moving being, projects that displace this truth with another, domineering way of being. From my discussion of puissance, we can say that the essence of truth is the compassionate freedom that lets beings be the beings that they are. I argued above that the essence of the being of the body is its puissance, which is 'coming to presence by moving (drawing-penetrating-absence-presence), which is itself essential, limitless, productive desire, which is the power of our essential relatedness to all existence.' Technology is a process that transforms the limitless freedom of our essential relatedness to being-as-a-whole, pragmatically directing that freedom of movement into usefulness. This is a transformation of the infinite meaning of being that transforms and delimits the possibilities of becoming. In technology, the intrinsic meaning of being is re-sourced according to extrinsic requirements. Movement is appreciated, reflected on, indeed pursued no longer for its intrinsic playful, carnal relatedness to all existence, but for the use that can be drawn from it.

In the 'environment,' that is a well-known phenomenon. Planners of the James Bay Hydro Electric project, for example, did not reflect on and care for the being of nature in accordance with the intrinsic meaning of nature coming to presence as streams of water, flora, and fauna, but saw it instead as a source of energy useful to Hydro Québec and its project of exchanging natural resources for capital. Likewise, in technologies of the body, an appreciation of the intrinsic, erotic meaning of movement gives way to the requirement that bodies function as efficient resources for capitalist production and consumption. Technology challenges the way in which we care for the body, pressing us as individuals and as a society to abandon its limitless freedom in favour of its technological production. The pouvoir of technology replaces our essential freedom with an essential usefulness.

The body, of course, has become a resource for many social projects. Speaking of the body's socio-cultural usefulness in general, Bryan Turner (1992), while not using the term 'resource,' says that in modern social systems the body has become 'the principal field of political and

cultural activity' (12). Shilling (1993), calling on the substantial literature that says that racism is a socio-cultural phenomenon that uses the
body for the creation of hierarchical social difference, describes how
the production of social inequalities resources the body (100–27).
Bourdieu (1984) has written on the education of bodily habits for the
embodied production of class differences. And Donna Haraway (1988)
has spoken of the body being resourced for the production of gender
(592). But most important to a theory of the resourcing of the body is
Michel Foucault.

My analysis of pouvoir focuses on a tight-knit progression in three
phases – subjection, which leads to body capital, which is the great
desideratum of body fascism.

Subjection

Foucault says that a mode of organization of the body has developed
in modernity that is qualitatively different from its predecessors. Rather
than being a repressive force located externally and inefficiently in the
power of the sovereign to seize life and possessions (1980, 135–42) and
make that power known by the public spectacle of sovereign power,
such as the practice of public executions (1979), in modernity (while
such external power continues to exist in the state apparatus) individuals wield that power internally – much more efficiently, meticu-
lously, and insidiously – on behalf of the power of social organization.
A special subjectivity has developed that diffuses power through the
life of the population. This has been a shift from the negative power of
seizure (of things, time, bodies, ultimately life itself) to the positive
power of the production of life.

One of the chief characteristics of modernity is the extent of human
control, both over nature in general and over humans in particular.
Foucault says that until the seventeenth century, the power exercised
over the population was haphazard and inefficient, dependent on the
intrusion of external authority in the lives of the people. With modernity, just as the power of production of goods was rationalized and
made vastly more efficient and capable of high levels of controlled
production, so too there were rationalizations of day-to-day life that
were geared to productivity and control – 'the controlled insertion of
bodies into the machinery of production and the adjustment of the
population to economic processes,' which Foucault calls 'biopower,' 'a
power whose highest function was perhaps no longer to kill, but to

invest life through and through' (1980, 141).[20] 'The old power of death that symbolized sovereign power was now carefully supplanted by the administration of bodies and the calculated management of life. During the classical period, there was a rapid development of various disciplines – universities, secondary schools, barracks, workshops; there was the emergence, in the field of political practices and economic observation, of the problems of birthrate, longevity, public health, housing, and migration. Hence there was an explosion of numerous techniques for achieving the subjugation of bodies and the control of populations, marking the beginning of the era of "biopower"' (140).

Foucault says that biopower takes two related forms: the body as a machine (i.e., 'the anatomo-politics of the human body') and the population as a controllable biological set of processes (i.e., 'the biopolitics of the population'). These metaphors and conceptual frameworks (which in chapter 3 I show to be fundamental to the scientific technology of physical fitness) are not just ways of *thinking* about the body; they are political dispositions towards the body that render it a useful resource. Biopower is not just a realm of *speculative* discourse – one interesting way among many of thinking about life, the body, and the possibilities for human life. Biopower sets about producing human life, organizing it socially and culturally, limiting the ways in which it may come to presence. As such, it is decidedly a political power.

In modernity an extensive 'government of the body' was cultivated as an 'indispensable element in the development of capitalism' (Foucault 1980, 141). Foucault speaks of this as the 'management of [the body's] forces.' He does not say what he means by the body's forces – although his *History of Sexuality* traces part of this administration through what he calls the 'uses of pleasure.' Pleasure, however, is just one facet of body force, one manifestation of the body's capacity for intensity (Deleuze and Guattari 1987, 154–5), or, in the language that I have developed here, pleasure is but one of the textures of puissance.[21] I suggest that the management of the body's forces is actually the resource management of its puissance. This is nothing less than the calculated extraction of its capacity to move and connect. Biopower organizes the movement of the body in the interests of social order for the maximization of capital production. It marshals the free play of puissance in the service of production and consumption, for which a high degree of social order and control is also necessary. To be highly productive (both as a producer of goods and images and as a consumer of the same – mass consumption being a form of economic activity in so far as mass consumption is the necessary corollary of mass production ([Featherstone 1991]), the body must move along prescribed paths. The body as (drawing-penetrating-absence-presence) comes to presence by being drawn into forms of absence that produce an economic social order. Another way of putting this is that modern desire (a mode of moving that serves social economics of consumer capitalism) desires paths that give presence to productivity, in terms either of the production of 'goods' (material, cultural, intellectual, spiritual, and so on) or of their consumption. This is desire that moves as a useful resource. It is desire that inserts the body's movement into the machinery of production and economic processes. The corollary is wasteful desire: desire that does not contribute to, or even undermines, production and consumption.

Similarly, Georges Bataille has considered the movement of desire in terms of productive and non-productive expenditure. Productive expenditure (of desire), he says, works within the logic of the balance sheet, wherein the expenditure must be commensurate with the purchase of life within the established structural and productive value-logics of the society. It should also be as parsimonious as possible, maximizing the culturally normative return on a particular expenditure of energy (of puissance, to use my term). Non-productive expenditure, in contrast, breaks out of the logic of the balance sheet and seeks no return on the expenditure of desire. Here, rather than expending puissance in order to gain normative cultural value, it does so precisely to lose such normative culture. Bataille's celebration of the notion of non-productive expenditure flies in the face of bourgeois productive respectability; rather than championing the accumulation of cultural wealth, it seeks its loss, and therefore the freedom of moving beyond, of transcending those logics.

Body Capital

Pierre Bourdieu has developed a sociological theory of the capitalization of the body. While he does not claim to have articulated a fully-fledged theory of the body in society (Shilling 1993, 128), his conceptualization of the commodification of physical capital enhances what I have been saying about the resourcing of the body in modern capitalism. Bourdieu (1978; 1984; 1988) points out that the body is commodified in three related ways: as labour power, as cultural symbol, and as social nexus. Shilling (1993) summarizes as follows:

Bourdieu's analysis of the body involves an examination of the multiple ways in which the body has become commodified in modern societies. This refers not only to the body's implication in the buying and selling of labour power, but to the methods by which the body has become a more comprehensive form of *physical capital*; a possessor of power, status and distinctive symbolic forms which is integral to the accumulation of various resources. The production of physical capital refers to the development of bodies in ways which are recognized as possessing value in social fields, while the conversion of physical capital refers to the translation of bodily participation in work, leisure, and other fields into different forms of capital. Physical capital [the body] is most usually converted into economic capital (money, goods and services), cultural capital (for example, education) and social capital (social networks which enable reciprocal calls to be made on the goods and services of its members). (127–8)

In modern society, the body is a commodity that has exchange value in (at least) several respects: It has the value of being able to perform work and thus be exchanged in the labour market. It has cultural value in its capacity for symbolic exchange – for instance, the symbolic value of the bodies of athletes (Hoberman 1984; 1994), of the hard, slim body of the 'physically fit' person (Bordo 1990), of the muscular body of the masculine man (Bordo 1993; Whitson 1994), of the empowered body of the muscular woman (Bolin 1992a; 1992b; 1992c; Markula 1995), of the ironic body of the gay man (Pronger 1992), as well as of the complex valuing and devaluing of bodies in the logics of racisms (Dyer 1997; Gladwell 1997; Goldberg 1990; 1993; Hodge 1990; hooks 1992). The body also has the social exchange value of tastes, needs, and habits that operate in the social exchange within and between social groups – consider, for instance, the immensely efficient systems of exchange of sexual pleasure in the commercialized gay male community (bars, bathhouses, backrooms, cinemas) of a city such as Toronto.

Bourdieu's conception of the commodification of the body can help us analyse the body's capital capacities in the technology of physical fitness in chapter 3. However, Bourdieu is not critical of the commodification of the body as such, as my analysis of the resourcing interplay of puissance and pouvoir attempts to be; instead, he focuses on the unequal opportunities afforded people in the hierarchical and privileging context of class for developing and benefiting from such commodification.[22]

Massumi (1992) points out that the commodification of life is now extensive and is at its fullest in high-technology capitalism, where

> the presence of the consumer/commodity axis of the capitalist relation [is operative] in every point of social space-time ... Everything can be bought, even life itself. There is a patent out on the human genome. A new mouse was just copyrighted. Whole species are now being bought and sold. Life forms are not simply captured by an external mechanism and put up for sale (as in the fur industry or trade of wild animals for pets); the very form of a life that has never existed in nature is commercialized at its point of emergence. It is captured from its future. The capitalist machine has developed perceptual abilities that enable it to penetrate life and direct its unfolding. It can go straight to the code of its molarity, resolve it into its constituents parts (in this case genes) [in the case of physical fitness, metabolism, for instance], recombine them to yield a special order product (adult individuals), and market the final product – or the transformational *process* itself [scientific regimens of physical fitness]. (133–4)

Deleuze and Guattari have also considered the development of capital in their theory of the body, specifically in the relations of puissance and pouvoir. Pre-capitalist desire, they say, was territorialized according to codes that named properties that were seen to be somehow 'inherent' to desire. Homosexual desire, for instance, was codified as inherently evil and subsequently reproduced in the binary logic of good and evil, salvation and damnation, and so on. Similarly the body is cast as inherently base, and the soul inherently lofty. Desire is thus directed and lived according to these codes. The free flow of desire is truncated by what is thought to be its inherent logic. Shades of Freud here – life without codes becomes terrifying: 'To code desire – and the fear, the anguish of decoded flows – is the business of the socius' (Deleuze and Guattari 1987, 139).[23] In this way the coding socius becomes the shelter, the caretaker of flows of desire that must be controlled.

Capitalism, say Deleuze and Guattari (1987), brings about a shift that frees desire from the tyranny of 'inherent' codes, but at great cost. 'Capitalism is the only social [system] that is constructed on the basis of decoded flows, substituting for intrinsic [inherent] codes an axiomatic of abstract quantities in the form of money. Capitalism therefore liberates the flows of desire, but under the social conditions that define its limit and the possibility of its own dissolution, so that it is constantly opposing with all its exasperated strength the movement that drives it toward this limit. At capitalism's limit the deterritorialized socius gives way to the body without organs, and the decoded flows throw themselves into desiring production. Hence [as Marx has taught us], it is correct to retrospectively understand all history in the light of capitalism' (139–40).

Capitalism recodifies desire in the quantitative abstraction of value. Everything under capitalism has more or less *value*. Capitalism frees desire of its 'inherent' codification in logics such as good and evil, only to recodify it according to various logics of value. Deleuze and Guattari say that valued desire – bodies as valuable – has organ-ized the body in such a way, codified it such, that desire reproduces the logics of value in the same way that a musical recording (especially a digital recording) reproduces only what the recording company wants! The properly socialized body may play only that which it has been coded to perform. Desire is thus played out, indeed produced, in a highly restricted way. Capitalism has freed the flow of desire (puissance) to such an extent that at the same time it must channel desire (pouvoir) so that the organization of capitalism is not undone (Deleuze and Guattari 1983, 22–36).[24] Capitalism operationalizes desire by translating it into the 'abstraction' of pure commodity exchange value. In a historical process, the body/desire that was traditionally defined and controlled by religious tradition in the 'inherent' dynamics of sin and purity, or by psychiatry's analysis of the 'inherent' drives of id and Oedipus, loses all intrinsic meaning.[25] Religion and psychiatry, according to Deleuze and Guattari (1983), constitute a despotic rule over desire, in the form of hermeneutic imperialisms that code the flows of desire in the contexts of religious or psychiatric meanings which they respectively claim to be inherent in the desire. Our BwO is thus socialized: 'The prime function incumbent upon the socius has always been to codify the flows of desire, to inscribe them, to record them, to see to it that no flow exists that is not properly dammed up, channelled, regulated' (33).

Capitalism is a social system that first and foremost resources desire, rather than simply repressing it. This happens in a historical (and indeed ongoing) process of freeing desire from its repression in despotic hermeneutics so that it is available to the marketplace – exchanged as easily and amorally as money. Reworking Marx on the contradictions of capital, Deleuze and Guattari observe that such free-

ing of desire tends towards the destruction of all social systems, including the capitalist one that set it free. While capitalism frees desire
to be a resource, it must concomitantly re-repress it in order to keep it
subjugated to the system and thus available as a resource. All in all,
Deleuze and Guattari say that this is a process of decoding and
deterritorializing the flows of desire that perpetuates itself by recoding
and reterritorializing desire. But freeing desire, they write, is always
dangerous to the socius, for some of it might escape the process of
recoding and reterritorializing that reins it in. This, as they argue at
great length in the two books on Capitalism and Schizophrenia, is
what produces schizophrenia, sexual 'perversions,' and other 'mon-
strous' social deviations (Massumi 1992, 93–142).

In this context, we can conceive puissance as the power of our decoded and deterritorialized BwO, and pouvoir as the power that
recodes and reterritorializes. Deleuze and Guattari (1983) write about
this relationship:

> The *capitalist machine* ... is faced with the task of decoding and
> deterritorializing the flows. Capitalism does not confront this situation
> from the outside, since it experiences it as the very fabric of its existence,
> as both its primary determinant and its *fundamental raw material* [the flow
> of desire or puissance as a resource], its form and its function, and delib-
> erately perpetuates it, in all its violence, with all the powers at its com-
> mand. Its sovereign production and repression can be achieved in no
> other way. Capitalism is in fact born of the encounter of two sorts of
> flows: the decoded flows of production in the form of money–capital,
> and the decoded flows of labour in the form of the 'free worker.' Hence,
> unlike previous social machines, the capitalist machine is incapable of
> providing a code that will apply to the whole of the social field. By
> substituting money for the very notion of a code, it has created an axiom-
> atic of abstract quantities that keeps moving further and further in the
> direction of the deterritorialization of the socius. Capitalism tends to-
> ward a threshold of decoding that will destroy the socius in order to
> make it a body without organs and unleash the flows of desire. (33,
> emphasis added)

Capitalism responds to the potential 'havoc' of free-flowing desire by
reterritorializing it:

> What we are really trying to say is that capitalism, through its process of
> production, produces an awesome schizophrenic accumulation of energy

or charge, against which it brings all its vast powers of repression to bear, but which nevertheless continues to act as capitalism's limit. For capitalism constantly counteracts, constantly inhibits this inherent tendency while at the same time allowing it free rein; it continually seeks to avoid reaching its limit while simultaneously tending toward that limit. Capitalism institutes or restores all sorts of residual and artificial, imaginary, or symbolic territories, thereby attempting, as best it can, to recode, to rechannel persons who have been defined in terms of abstract quantities. The more the capitalist machine deterritorializes, decoding and axiomatizing flows in order to extract surplus value from them, the more its ancillary apparatuses, such as government bureaucracies and the forces of law and order, do their utmost to reterritorialize. (34–5)

The plight of the body in consumer culture offers a particularly good example of the process of deterritorializing and reterritorializing desire. The ideal consumer is a hedonist, succumbing to desire, eating, drinking, pursuing sex, running marathons for fun, and so on, expressing the freedom of desire in the 'vast' supermarket of consumer 'choice.' But maintenance of such hedonism requires individuals' subjection to the socio-economic system that keeps them employed and capable of purchasing the products that help them to release desire, thus creating what Bordo (1990, 201) calls a contradictory personality structure, or what Crawford (1984, 90) describes as managed desire. This is the repressive force not only of having to return to work after a weekend of 'debauchery,' but more problematically of being coerced into following restricted channels of 'free-wheeling' desire: i.e., commodified forms of experience that are available in the marketplace and within the realm of 'normal' desire. This restriction of desire is a process in which the codifying interests of managing human capital resources appropriate the free flow of energy. This kind of desire, I suggest, is fascist.

Body Fascism

I am using 'fascist' in the same sense as Foucault does in his description of Deleuze and Guattari's work – 'not only historical fascism, the fascism of Hitler and Mussolini – which was able to mobilize and use the desire of the masses so effectively – but also the fascism in us all, in our heads and in our everyday behaviour, the fascism that causes us to love power, to desire the very thing that dominates and exploits us' (Foucault 1983, xiii). Mark Seem (1983) problematizes the popularity and insidiousness of fascism similarly: 'Everybody wants to be a fascist. Deleuze and Guattari want to know how these beliefs succeed in taking hold of a body, thereby silencing the productive machines of the libido' (xx).

And so by fascism I mean the desire to order, organ-ize, control, repress, direct, impose limits – to interrupt the free flow of puissance and subordinate it to pouvoir. Fascism crystallizes in the popular desire to be led, to be the subject of power. So this fascism is a *will* within us to desire, albeit often unwittingly, a life of domination. Foucault, much like Adorno and others of the Frankfurt School, asked how a population co-operates so well with fascist projects. The answer, he says, lies in the ways in which the force relations of power produce our desires. Deleuze and Guattari also address this, commenting that our desire is produced in spheres of recodification – for example, in consuming a range of products in the consumer marketplace, in expressing 'normal' or, for that matter, 'abnormal' desire, or in making a certain kind of body (fit, productive, marketable). So pouvoir, at work in the body, reproducing a record of subjected desire, is body fascism.

The label 'fascist' is very strong, loaded with emotion, evocative of the worst manifestations of humanity, of the ugliest expressions of life in the twentieth century. Rebecca Comay (1995) warns against minimizing the horrors of the historical fascism of the mid-twentieth century – specifically German fascism, which saw the brutal repression and murder of millions of people. She critiques a misconception that understands fascism as a universal element of the human condition, our sinful estate. Presciently, she notes the 'risk [of] recycling generalized theories of "totalitarianism" which would relativize the specificity of fascism as a historical phenomenon ... [which] would dissolve the threat of fascism by occluding its specific material determinations. Explaining everything and therefore nothing, the theory of fascism's ghosts would all too easily evaporate its object within the comfortable paranoia of a universal phantomology ... Everywhere and nowhere, spooky, disembodied, fascism would thus become a consoling bogeyman, alluring, enchanting, arousing aesthetic thrills and therefore safely rehabilitated within the economy of the sublime' (3).

I am not suggesting that fascism is universal in the human condition or saying that the historical specifics of German fascism did not create a particularly heinous reality. Indeed, I base my use of the word 'fascism' in the material history of capitalism as an authoritarian force that aims to resource the essential freedom of the body and to transform the possibilities for being human. Fascism has various techniques – the flagrant brutality of Auschwitz was one of them; the hidden nihilism of pouvoir is another. They are both profound negations of the freedom of our BwO, of our potential for wholeness. The fascism of Hitler and Mussolini is a kind of crude fascism, resorting to jackboots, torture, and murder in order to gain its regime repressively. The fascism that I am describing is more 'sophisticated.' European fascism of the 1930s and 1940s incarcerated and abused millions of people and in so doing attempted to crush the spirit of the continent. But it did so at great cost – its ostentatious display forced resistance. The fascism of the modern technological project achieves, as Foucault would say, great controlling power at very low cost: the lack of bloodshed, the almost invisible hand of this power, leads to little chance of rebellion. The 'positive' (productive rather than repressive) nature of this fascism makes it attractive to the subjected and requires little more than the promise of success within its system to get people participating wholeheartedly.

But is it not unfair to label aspects of almost everyone's everyday life – the research of honest scientists, as well as a tradition of physical education – with this loaded word? No. For just as critical theorists gave us pause to think about the insidiousness of ideology, as, not dissimilarly, Freud invited us to consider the terrifying motives of the socially constructed unconscious, and as feminists noted the omnipresence of the patriarchal construction of reality, so too Heidegger, Foucault, and Deleuze ask us to look in to the darkness of our modern technological souls. Fascism is a form of totalitarianism – the total subjection of humanity to the political imperatives of systems whose concern is their own productivity, not flourishing, enlightening, plateaux of intensities of Being. 'Fascism' is not too strong a word, because the phenomenon at work here is not a cursory imposition on the way in which we are expected to go about our lives, an occasional oppression, exploitation that takes place just on the surface of human experience. This phenomenon is more than the unwelcome appropriation of *bits* of life. It is the production of life that seeks nothing less than complete identity with pouvoir.

It goes, therefore, beyond Marx's critique of the alienation of workers in the labour process and of the ideological apparatuses that assist in that process. For alienation presupposes at least a duality between an essentially free human being and the appropriation of his or her work in the service of capital – the image of the beautiful creature, chained, is the image of the alienated worker. The fascism of which I speak here attempts not to chain a naturally free essence. It *makes* us fascist. According to Adorno and Horkheimer (1972), fascism is the last stage in the 'logic of decay' inherent in the human species itself. 'The process of civilization took the form of a spiral of increasing reification which was set in motion by the original acts of subjugating nature and reached its logical conclusion in fascism' (Honeth 1993). This concept of civilization denies any modernist notion of progress, except as manifest in the intensification of the forces of production. Similarly, the identity of pouvoir and fascism that I am proposing here is progressive only in the sense of intensifying the forces of production and consumption. So the use of this loaded term, 'fascist,' is appropriate precisely because the phenomenon that it signifies is loaded.

Moreover, the point of critiques of fascism, such as those of Adorno, those of Deleuze and Guattari, and my modest attempt here, is to open the possibilities of living outside fascism. Foucault says in his preface to Deleuze and Guattari's *Anti-Oedipus* (1983a) that the work is 'an introduction to the Non-Fascist Life,' the objective of which is to 'counter all forms of fascism, whether already present or impending.' This endeavour requires 'the tracking down of all varieties of fascism, from the enormous ones that surround and crush us to the petty ones that constitute the tyrannical bitterness of our everyday lives' (Foucault 1983a, xiii, xiv).

Deleuze and Guattari's theory of the power of capitalism to use the body by removing its 'inherent' codes (for example, as the temple of the Holy Spirit or a source of evil passions) and to 'free' it to the abstractions of monetary value shows how desire becomes a resource for capitalist production, especially in 'late' consumer capitalism (Jameson 1984). It also reveals how desire can become a waste product by virtue of the same system that produces it as a resource – for example, in the lack of economic productivity of schizophrenics, drug and sex 'addicts,' and some athletes such as 'surf bums.' And capitalism's 'ancillary apparatuses, such as government bureaucracies and the forces of law and order [are doing] their utmost to reterritorialize' (Deleuze and Guattari 1983, 35) the body by empowering the institutions and professions of the police, medicine, health promotion, and physical fitness to rein in desire where it 'gets out of hand,' arresting those in possession of 'illicit' drugs, medicalizing them, and coercing them into 'health' with physical fitness routines, for instance. But reterritorialization includes much more than institutional repression following on too much freedom.

Reterritorialization is productive. Following Foucault's productive theory of power, which is not a departure from Deleuze and Guattari, I suggest that reterritorialization occurs where desire is channelled (Deleuze and Guattari's own term), specifically where the economic logic of resource and waste management produces desire. Here is the cultural imperative for desire either to produce itself in terms of its overall economic utility (a resource) or accept a marginalized life as a 'waste.' (It is worth noting here that modernity's waste may well become postmodernity's source of resistance, as Bataille, Deleuze and Guattari, Massumi, and numerous queer theorists suggest *celebrating* and *pursuing* the 'wasteful' life of the margins of productivity.) Either puissance is rendered useful to pouvoir, or it is cast aside. This is not the controlled desire of Weber's asceticism or Elias's civilizing process; it is desire transformed as essentially useful to power. Here is puissance giving pouvoir the power of life.

Fascist culture does not *replace* the power of life (puissance) with the power of government (pouvoir); rather, pouvoir *achieves* puissance in fascist desire. Pouvoir produces puissance as pouvoir, and puissance gives pouvoir its puissance. In fascism, life and government are one and the same. Fascism is complete where the power of life (puissance) can reflect on itself in its essential freedom – a freedom that I attempted to invoke in my discussion of puissance above – *only* as it is useful to governmentality. Here is the great danger that Heidegger says lurks in the modern technological mode of being (Heidegger 1938; 1953; 1954). It is, arguably, a turning point in history that may have already occurred, inextricably tying humans and the ecosphere to the nihilism of a fascist destiny.

Pouvoir then is a fascist government of the body that produces useful desire, a way of moving/being that is essentially economic. Pouvoir can be conceptualized in my analysis of the body as the moving event of being (above) as resourcing puissance by insinuating itself in the structure of puissance as drawing-penetrating-absence-presence. Pouvoir appropriates the absential space that in puissance draws presence into itself (an intrinsic and essentially free meaning structure) and instead charts the course by which desire comes to presence as a resource (an extrinsic and essentially subjugated meaning structure).[26] Rather than compassionately opening a limitless freedom for becoming – which is the authentic work of empty desire –

absence, through pouvoir, draws presence into usefulness, a limited manner of coming to presence, whose logos is not intrinsic, reflective freedom and attunement to being-as-a-whole (the essence of being as movement), but is rather the extrinsic technological logos of economic utility, which determines useful and useless desire.

The channelling, directing, coercive power of pouvoir closes the reflective opening of being that is absence. The wonder of absence is the opening of the infinite potential for becoming, which Deleuze and Guattari call our 'undifferentiated BwO.' Puissance is our potential for infinite connectivity. Pouvoir marshals the limitless power of absence, which is the opening of the infinity of being, and constructs instead a limited, finite path. The erasure of our infinity is the nihilistic heart of fascism. The nihilistic acceptance, indeed enthusiastic pursuit, of finite ways of life represents the triumph of fascism in everyday life. Heidegger says that 'nihilism is the age in which [the infinity] of Being has become a vapour, a vacuous abstraction, "nothing at all"' (Caputo 1986, 185). Under pouvoir, absence opens presence, but it is the opening of nihilism, which of course is ultimately closure.

Produced by pouvoir, desire becomes the powerful autogenous force by which the body brings itself to presence essentially as a resource. The ethical problem here is that pouvoir, by resourcing desire, evacuates it of its intrinsic freedom and essential relatedness. Pouvoir, productively resourcing puissance, aggressively marshals the intrinsic meaning of the body, effectively making extrinsic meaning intrinsic. In short, the body is technologized, becoming essentially a resource, brought to presence in its use-value. Under pouvoir, desire is therefore free only in so far as it functions within the economics of usefulness, participating in production and consumption. Desire's freedom as a resource is the 'virtual' freedom of consumer choice and career planning – a far cry from the freedom of puissance.[27]

Rendered useful by pouvoir, desire's puissance – its erotic power of connection – is transformed. Pouvoir makes connections, but they are functional and rendered meaningful in the parergonal logic of use-value. Pouvoir is not just the production of resources; it is also the dividing up of reality into resources and waste products. This is the element that Alderman adds to Heidegger's critique of modern technology – the productive transformation of what is into useful and useless being. Here is a parergonal logic that separates not only individual bodies into categories of useful and useless, but also some dimensions of the body as useful to the enframing of technology and other dimensions as second. The way in which this process is internalized is particularly interesting. And it marks a difference between the resourcing of 'nature' and the resourcing of desire. Strip mining, as an example of modern management of natural resources, is an aggressive transformation of the wilderness, as it were by an external force: industrial, technological man. Pouvoir's resourcing of desire, in contrast, is internal. Desire produces itself as a resource (as though the wilderness strip mined itself). It does this by making useful and useless paths of desire. Desire that does not contribute to the economics of production and consumption is useless, the wasted power of movement. So the development of paths of desire that allow it to render itself (the body) a useful resource is strategic to the success of pouvoir as a resourcing of the body. This is a crucial point: pouvoir is not an accomplished fact, but an ongoing process of resource production.

The relationship between puissance and pouvoir is itself a power relation, which is first and foremost an ongoing process, not a *fait accompli*. Foucault, from whose theory of biopower I am borrowing heavily, is often criticized for offering an overly determined theory of the body, the argument being that a body produced entirely in discourse is a body without agency, a body purely dominated. Toby Miller (1993) counters this critique: 'Foucault is quite explicit that he understands a prevailing *epistēmē* to be "a space of *dispersion*"' that is discontinuous and relatively open. It is not a "sovereign, unique and constraining form." The epistēmē is instead to be seen as a "complex relationship of successive displacements," not something moving toward a grand synthesis or "syncopated transcendental"' (175–6). For Foucault, power is always a *process*: 'Power must be understood in the first instance as the multiplicity of force relations, immanent in the sphere in which they operate and which constitute their own organization; as the process which, through ceaseless struggles and confrontations transforms, strengthens, or reverses them; as the support which these force relations find in one another, thus forming a chain or a system, or on the contrary, the dysfunctions and contradictions which isolate them from one another; and lastly as the strategies in which they take effect, whose general design or institutional crystallization is embodied in the state apparatus, in the formulation of the law, in the various social hegemonies' (Foucault 1980a, 92–3).

The body understood as a dynamic, ongoing event of coming to presence in both its intrinsic puissance and its extrinsic pouvoir happens as a process of multiple force relations. In the first place this multiplicity involves the infinite interplay between puissance (as the intrinsic, playful, free, limitless, productive desire in its essential relatedness to all existence) and pouvoir (as the extrinsic government of the usefulness of desire). This multiplicity generates the power of modern human being. There are, of course, other force relations that I am not developing here but that also are central to the production of the modern body – notably, the multiple force relations of race, class, gender, physical (dis)ability, regionalism, linguistic heritage, and so on that support or undermine the economic resourcing of the body, which is the central concern of this book.[28]

Because the body is a moving event, these force relations take place in an ongoing process. This is a process that, through the 'ceaseless struggles and confrontations' of puissance and pouvoir, supports the modern technology of the body, 'thus forming a chain or a system, or on the contrary, the dysfunctions and contradictions which isolate them from one another.' Deleuze and Guattari have thematized this supportive interplay, arguing that while pouvoir (as resourcing capitalism) seeks to exploit puissance for the production of capital, it creates freedoms (sometimes momentary, sometimes virtually permanent) that can escape its regulating grasp – in, for example, schizophrenic experience, playing with recreational drugs, sexual outlawlessnes, and rave culture (Jordan 1995). My experience that I wrote about in the first pages of this book – swimming to develop physical capital and simultaneously finding transcendence – was and continues to be a partial and modest but enlightening escape from the grasp of pouvoir. And finally, 'the *strategies* in which they take effect, whose general design or institutional crystallization is embodied in the state apparatus, in the formulation of the law, in the various social hegemonies' are the various programs for making technological desire.

Biopower, Foucault points out, operates in two basic forms, which are mutually supportive of each other: one produces the individual body as a machine, an 'anatomo-politics of the human body,' and the other deals with 'regulatory controls: a biopolitics of the population.' The latter focuses on the biological processes of the body in terms of controlling 'propagation, births and mortality, the level of health, life expectancy and longevity, with all the conditions that can cause these to vary' (Foucault 1980a, 139). These regulatory controls of the population's biological processes serve the interests of keeping the individual body functioning biologically well as a machine as well as of controlling the larger population's biological processes so that it serves the disciplinary needs of the capitalist socio-economic system, which requires ever-greater 'efficiencies.' In other words, they direct the movement of the body both individually and collectively. They do so through the canny intertwinings of discipline and knowledge. Discipline, says Foucault (1979), is the political technology of the body that makes individuals useful (26, 211) and controls human multiplicities. The body cannot be a useful resource when it effectively resists being one; desire cannot be harnessed and developed if it is not available as a resource. When the body is coerced into presence primarily, if not exclusively, in terms of its utility, it is rendered docile.

Integral to making the body docile and thus useful is the conception of the body as intelligible – that is, the body is rendered useful by the manner in which it is known. Here is the intimate connection of knowledge and power about which Foucault speaks and that formed the basis of much of the theory of science that I outlined above. As the philosophy of the limit reveals, the paradigms of systems of knowledge determine what is seen and thus what becomes real. In my theory of the body, this becomes a matter of paradigms (specifically, the power play of puissance and pouvoir) determining what the systems of knowledge of the body see and the realities that they set out to produce.

Conclusion: Body and Transcendence

The relations of pouvoir and puissance are relations of domination and subordination, which make the body's energy, its power to move, which is its be-ing, available to the modern projects of docile human production and consumption. This dynamic of domination ensnares essential human freedom in the modern technological project of resource management, mined for the energy that it makes available to the economics of production and consumption. As Foucault argues through much of his work, knowledge of the body is crucial to maximizing its usefulness. In chapter 3, I examine the ways in which the technology of physical fitness codes the body in order to make it useful to the modern technological project.

But these relations of dominance and submission have their ironic subversive potentials as well. The life of domination cannot be overcome by instituting new regimes of domination, replacing one set of codes with another, one regime with another. What is necessary is the transcendence of domination itself. The puissance of the moving body, I suggest, offers such potential for transcendence. Puissance, I have been saying, is the life-giving power of opening, the gift (*Es gibt*) of absence in drawing-penetrating-absence-presence. That life-giving gift is fullest when it is empty – the freest space of movement is an empty, unstructured, uncoded, deterritorialized space. Emptiness (*sunyata*) is the clearing of space in the movement of life that transcends ego and the other social constructions of the self (Glass 1995). Moving in emptiness, the body moves beyond the territorializations of pouvoir. Emptiness deterritorializes the body's social construction.

From a personal, psychological perspective, the working of emptiness cleaves the homogeneous surface of the self and opens the abyss. The abyss poses a deep threat to the self, because it empties the codes that construct the self, that organize the body in the socio-economic scheme of things. As Deleuze and Guattari point out, deterritorialization is a process of becoming different. Openness to radical difference, to living life in the open regions, in alterity, is the ethical quest of the philosophy of the limit – to be open to living with/in that which is outside the system. The giving power of puissance is its openness. The reflective or meditative practice of emptiness makes it possible to live compassionately in that openness without attachment to the territorializations that have constructed the self. That open region, allowed to be fully empty, is empty of codes, of language, and is therefore unnameable, unspeakable. Emanuel Levinas alludes to this quality as 'illeity.' '"Illeity" links up with "Other," "Infinite," and "Alterity" to form a metonymic chain of signifiers intended to evoke what cannot be designated' (Taylor 1987, 204). Being unspeakable, illeity leaves only a trace in discourse; certainly, it is not present in the words that I am using to allude to it on this page. In reflective movement, however, this mysterious, infinite, other announces itself in the clearing of the gerundive opening of drawing-penetrating-presence-absence. It remains unspeakable, but its trace can inform life in the most profound way.

PART TWO:
TEXTS AND PROCEDURES

3

The Texts of the Technology
of Physical Fitness

To begin with, there was the scale of the control: it was a question not of treating the body, en masse, 'wholesale,' as if it were an indisociable unity, but of working it 'retail,' individually; of exercising upon it a subtle coercion, of obtaining holds upon it at the level of the mechanism itself – movements, gestures, attitudes, rapidity: an infinitesimal power over the active body. Then there was the object of the control: it was not or was no longer the signifying elements of behaviour or the language of the body, but the economy, the efficiency of movements, their internal organization; constant bears upon the forces rather than upon the signs; the only truly important ceremony [for power] is that of exercise.

Michel Foucault 1979, 136–7

Naturalistic understandings of the technology of physical fitness accept it as a (mostly) scientifically informed way of optimizing the body's potential for health, productivity, longevity, and happiness. The object of this book is to show that there is more to the technology of physical fitness than the naturalistic reading appreciates. In the Introduction I mentioned the scholarly literature that is critical of aspects of physical fitness for supporting contradictions in the welfare state and contributing to its disciplinary apparatus, for playing an ideological role for the reproduction of class and gender, and for its patriarchally founded positivism, which has contributed to professional monopolies that marginalize women and others. In chapter 1 I drew together a political philosophy of science that shows ways in which science is not merely a (more or less) accurate, objective representation of reality but is actually deeply engaged in the highly political production of reality. And in chapter 2, I sketched a theory of the body that attempts to show how the body is open to technological discourses that exploit and limit the fulness of its potential. In this and the next chapters I draw together the theories of the body and of science from chapters 1 and 2 and attempt to show specifically how the science and technology of physical fitness set out to construct the body along fascist lines.

But at the outset, I want to make clear what I am not saying. I am not saying that regular physical activity, careful diet, and other disciplines of the body are necessarily bad. Regular physical activity and moderation in the expression of the desire for food, drink, and other pleasures can probably increase the functional capacity of the human 'organism.' As a very physically active person, I find great pleasure and a deep sense of well-being in physical exercise. And as a university teacher of the philosophy of physical education, I believe in the importance of a physical education. I am, however, critical of the dominant discourses of physical education and fitness. My critique here is analogous to the critical sociology of sport, which suggests that while one can engage in a sport and can gain skills that help one play the game better, learning a sport is never a purely technical matter. For when one is learning the technical skills of a sport one can at the same time in the same setting – depending on how the sport culture is structured – learn, internalize, and operationalize oppressive cultural discourses, such as classism, racism, sexism, heterosexism, and homophobia. In that non-uncommon situation, sport becomes much more than a simple game of physical skill; it is an institutionalized indoctrination into living a classist, racist, sexist, and homophobic life. As writers often say in the history and sociology of sport: sport is *not* just a game. In a similar vein, I seek to show that the technology of physical fitness is not just a simple matter of analysing the body and suggesting strategies for improving physiological and psychological function. The analysis below attempts to reveal the full cultural implications of what the science and technology of physical fitness attempt to produce. The problem, then, is not with physical activity per se, but with the modern technological production of it.

How does the technology of physical fitness figure in the dynamics of pouvoir and puissance? I suggest that it territorializes puissance by producing texts that construct an implicit soteriology – i.e., a doctrine of salvation – for the modern subject within the parergonal logic of modern technology, which is aggressive resource management. We can see versions of the doctrine first in the position papers, the policy statements on health, and the physical fitness initiatives of government agencies. Second, versions appear in the scientific papers, textbooks, and manuals of academic exercise science. Third, the doctrine also circulates in popular books, magazines, and video tapes on exercise and physical fitness. Fourth, physical fitness appraisal, exercise prescriptions, regimens, procedures, equipment and exercise, and diet log books articulate this doctrine as well. And, fifth, popular representations of the fit body abound.

Together these five elements form the 'intertextual ensemble' that shapes the technological culture of physical fitness. This ensemble creates a framework for the production of desire – via description, inscription, and prescription (see chapter 4) – for those who come into contact with it, and especially for those who follow disciplinary ways of life in accordance with the doctrine. These texts enframe desire by establishing a *logos*, a hermeneutic circle, that attempts to circumscribe how we understand the body and ultimately how it should live. These texts give the body meaning and therefore direction in accordance with the parergonal logic of their implicit doctrine of salvation. This soteriology, I suggest, comes out of one of the central myths of modern Western patriarchal culture.

Before deconstructing the technology of physical fitness in chapter 4, I wish to trace the shape of the five types of texts that represent its project for the body. Some of these 'texts' are such in the most traditional sense; they exist as words on the pages of books, journals, manuals, and advertisements. Some, as visual representations, are also texts in so far as they can be 'read' for their content. And others – the social practices of the technology of physical fitness, such as following a particular exercise regimen – can also be read as texts, in that they inscribe and prescribe ways of living. Indeed, as Derrida has argued, the several-thousand-year legacy of Western culture is founded on the primacy of the word and a host of complex inscribing practices that profoundly limit the realm of the possible. Inscription is fundamental to the Western ability to see and understand. This is the 'as structure' of Western ways of perceiving that I discussed in chapter 2; we conceive things as they appear in the logocentric traditions that we have inherited (Derrida 1978; Cornell 1992; Sheehan 1983, 137). In that way tradition inscribes reality.

The 'truth' of an inscription therefore 'arises out of the interlocking relations of the textually conceived system as their effect, producing in turn, effects of behaviour, emotion, power, within the signifying terms of the system' (Radloff 1993, 639). The 'truth' of the texts of the technology of physical fitness is an effect of the technology's inscribing practices. Put simply, becoming physically fit by heeding the directions of the texts on physical fitness is an effect of the texts. This might seem to be merely stating the obvious. But what is crucial here is that *the authenticity of 'being a physically fit person' is the effect of the parergonal logic of the underlying soteriology of physical fitness, as it is realized in the textual practices of the technology.* Textual, inscribing practices code the body and direct desire, and pouvoir resources and (re)territorializes puissance. The technology of physical fitness is a logocentric enterprise.

From Bernhard Radloff, I take the following broad definition of 'text': 'A text is a structure composed of elements of signification by which the greater or lesser unity of those elements makes itself manifest. A text comprises, consequently, elements of signification, the unity of these elements and the manifestation of this unity. In narrower usages "text" is restricted to linguistic unities, in wider usages any group of phenomena, and even being itself, may be understood as a "text"' (Radloff 1993, 639). My deconstructive task in this chapter therefore is to consider the ways in which the texts of the technology of physical fitness manifest particular unities of signification that limit and exploit the puissance of desire.

The formation of knowledge of the body in these texts is productive of ways of life. As Foucault (1979) observes:

Power and knowledge directly imply one another; there is no power relation without the correlative constitution of a field of knowledge, nor any knowledge that does not presuppose and constitute at the same time power relations. These 'power-knowledge relations' are to be analysed, therefore, not on the basis of a subject of knowledge who is or is not free in relation to the power system, but, on the contrary, the subject who knows the objects to be known and the modalities of knowledge must be regarded as so many effects of these fundamental implications of power-knowledge and their historical transformations. In short, it is not the activity of the subject of knowledge that produces a corpus of knowledge, useful or resistant to power, but power-knowledge, the processes and struggles that traverse it and of which it is made up, that determines the forms and possible domains of knowledge. (27–8)

My deconstruction of the texts of the technology of physical fitness attempts to show what kind of subjectivity the inscription of these texts makes possible in pouvoir's resourcing of puissance.

The focus of this analysis is on physical fitness. There are certainly significant intersections between the cultures of physical fitness and of competitive sport, especially in so far as the technologies employed produce the subjected body/desire that I describe in the next chapter. But a full analysis of competitive sport using the theories of science and the body that I developed in chapters 1 and 2 would constitute a sizeable monograph in its own right. So while the competitive athletic body shares much in common with the physically fit body that I am deconstructing here, I defer to another volume consideration of the intersections between competitive sports cultures and the technology of physical fitness.

I limit my discussion in this chapter to the texts of modern Western and Northern cultures. A wealth of texts on the body and training lies outside this tradition – the texts of yoga, tai chi, tantrism, akido, tai-kwon do, and so on. There are also Southern traditions of bodily training, as well as North American Native, that are less well known to the West. And there is a small minority of Western texts on the body that focus on body awareness, often referred to as somatics, that do not follow the modern technological trajectory that I am analysing in this chapter. Such alternative texts could help foster the alterity to which I allude in the Postscript.

These five textual fields, because they work together as a disciplinary technology for the production of life, are profoundly interdependent. While the account below moves from government policies through academic science and through training manuals and techniques to popular representations of the fit body, it would be a mistake to understand this as a simple, hierarchical causal sequence – i.e., that government policy spawned scientific research, which informed training techniques that have made possible the popular image of the fit body. In chapter 1, I said that a political philosophy of science shows how scientific knowledge is embedded in a host of socio-cultural discourses; it both forms these discourses and is informed by them. And in chapter 2 I argued that nature, technology, science, and culture are intertwined. These textual fields cannot therefore be understood in a simple hierarchy. I hope that my deconstruction of the intertextual ensemble, following this more-or-less-simple summary of each textual field, shows how this is the case.

Government Policies and Publications

Academic and state interest in physical fitness is expressed in research and policies for preventive health care, which is often known as 'health promotion,' specifically as an aspect of 'lifestyle management.' Many proponents view health promotion as expressing a break with established perspectives on health, which conceptualize health in terms more of curing the sick than of maintaining and preserving health by identifying the social determinants of health and focusing on 'population health' and 'healthy communities.' Indeed, its champions see health promotion as a new anti-establishment paradigm, which is bringing to health administration and industry a major paradigm shift (Kickbusch 1994; Rootman and O'Neill 1994). Some proponents of health promotion trace its roots to the feminist and environmental movements (Kickbusch 1994, 8), implying that that demonstrates its anti-establishment roots. Other feminist accounts of health promotion, however, do not see it as being allied with the emancipatory impetus of feminism, but see it as more closely resembling the controlling culture operative in the marketing of consumer goods (Grace 1991). Proponents have tried very hard to make health promotion the established health paradigm. State support attests to the growing establishment of the discourse.

The state's endorsement of health promotion is important. By channelling funds and administrative support to research and implementation strategies, the government of Canada, like the governments of many other 'developed' countries, has put political weight behind a concept of health and human behaviour. Health promotion is thus not *just* a concept, just one philosophy of the body, life, and human behaviour among others; it is part of a Canadian program to govern people's bodies. By embracing health promotion, the government of Canada wants to change the way in which people live.

The operative medical definition of 'health' traditionally has revolved around the notion of the absence of disease (Rootman and Raeburn 1994, 57). Increasingly, the definition is being expanded to include other parameters. Medical and related physiological concepts of health focus on the state of an individual. *Black's Medical Dictionary* says: 'The state of health implies much more than freedom from disease, and good health may be defined as the attainment and maintenance of the highest state of mental and bodily vigour of which a person is capable' (MacPherson 1992, 265). The exercise physiologist Roy Shephard confirms this individual focus in his report on the Consensus Conference to the American Academy of Kinesiology and Physical Education in 1994, in which he expands on the official definition: 'A comprehensive approach would require consideration of such indices as health-related fitness, both acute temporary and more permanent chronic disabilities, absenteeism, overall social productivity, and the *individual's* demand for all types of medical services' (Shephard 1994, 289, emphasis added).

In contrast to the individualism of medical and physiological definitions of health stands a more social, indeed environmental, conceptualization. This was first officially stated by the World Health Organization (WHO) in 1947: 'Health is a state of complete physical, mental, and social well-being and not merely the absence of disease and infirmity' (Rootman and Raeburn 1994, 58). The WHO expanded the definition in 1986 to include an ecological dimension (World Health Organization 1986). The expanded definition is ecological in the sense that individuals, their families, society, and the environment comprise a whole that may or may not be healthy. Out of that comes notions such as 'healthy cities'[1] – i.e., whole urban environments that promote health in a variety of ways: socially, culturally, individually, in terms of the physical environment, as well as providing adequate health care and social support. As we see below, the technology of physical fitness does not draw on an ecology of health, focusing instead solely on individual physical and psychological health.

While health promotion was first formally recognized in Canada with the establishment of the Ontario Board of Health in 1882, it was not until publication of the Lalonde Report, *A New Perspective on the Health of Canadians* (Lalonde 1974), that health promotion garnered any serious government attention. Most government money for health, in the form of transfer payments to provincial ministries of health (the British North America Act, 1867, placed responsibility for health and welfare in the provincial domain), went to the medical treatment of disease. But by the end of the 1960s skyrocketing costs of medical care had become a concern. Numerous reports (including Canada 1969; 1973; Ontario 1974) called for a shift to less expensive forms of health care, which would stress health promotion and disease prevention. The current official rationale for government interest in health promotion is containment of health costs (Pederson, O'Neill, and Rootman 1994; Pinder 1988; 1994; Rootman and Raeburn 1994). In 1998 the government of Ontario, for example, justified a program called 'Active Ontario,' which is meant to increase physical activity in homes, workplaces, schools, recreational facilities, and health care programs, by arguing that the province could save $31 million annually on health care (http://www.activeontario.org/backgrounder.cfm).

Even before the appearance of the Lalonde Report, professional promoters of physical fitness had gathered for a National Conference on Fitness and Health in 1972. It produced twenty-four recommendations. Recommendation no. 1 calls for a 'comprehensive educational and promotional program of physical fitness and health' to 'motivate' Canadians 'into changing their living habits.' The recommendations focus on way of life and on the provision of tests and services that would 'motivate' people to do so. Recommendation no. 2 asks Recreation Canada to 'seek the cooperation of established "professional behaviour modification agents" and agencies who could provide expertise in changing the value system of Canadians, related to physical fitness' (Canada 1972, 124).

And the conference encouraged the government to use every means possible to encourage individuals to change their lives and their 'living habits' and 'values.' That included mass marketing campaigns (one of them was called 'Participaction'), widespread fitness testing of individuals, and harnessing the technological expertise of 'professional behaviour modification agents.' The current Canadian Physical Activity Fitness and Lifestyle Appraisal (CPAFLA) continues this focus on attempting to control the way in which individuals live and think about themselves. As in Canada, so governments throughout the modernized world have encouraged research on physical fitness and developed policies on health promotion through physical fitness.

In 1986 the government of Canada sponsored the Canadian Summit on Fitness. In the fourteen years since the National Conference on Fitness and Health, the majority of citizens had still not become active enough to affect their health and reduce medical costs: only one-third were considered even moderately active; only 10 per cent exercised at a level deemed by the American College of Sports Medicine (ACSM) to be sufficient to improve cardiovascular health; and of those who did begin a fitness program, 50 per cent dropped out during the first three to six months, which is often referred to as recidivism – a criminological term, interestingly enough. The summit in 1986 promoted a less rigorous approach, which it called 'Active Living,' arguing that lower and less consistent levels of physical activity, such as walking, gardening, and cleaning house, could also be beneficial to health.

The federal government has largely endorsed this approach in its propaganda on physical fitness. Bercovitz (1996) points out that while physiological studies did not for the most part find significant gains from such lower levels of exercise, the government continued to promote 'Active Living' in the hope that it would at least save some money. The CPAFLA prescribes 'active living' for those who are not already engaged in a rigorous fitness program and who seem unlikely to do so. It encourages those who have been doing less rigorous exercise, however, to do more. 'Active Living' is a concept promoted to incorporate into it those who resist the culture of physical fitness.

Scientific Texts

Over the last forty years, the growth of the sciences of physical fitness (biomechanics, exercise physiology, and psychology) has been substantial. The major medical research index (*Index Medicus*, which online is now called *Medline*) indicates that the number of times the words 'exercise,' 'exertion,' and 'physical activity' appeared as subjects in scientific journals increased from 1,090 in 1966 to 6,444 in 1998, with a total during that thirty-two-year period of 116,749.[2] These texts constitute an academic discourse on the technology of physical fitness. That technology is both the cultural context for the scientific discourse on fitness and the socio-cultural means for insinuating that discourse in the day-to-day production of modern life.

The texts of the exercise sciences assume a fairly simple, modernist, progressive, and cumulative concept of scientific knowledge. Knowledge of the body, physical activity, and health has progressed from the unsophisticated musings of Galen in the third century of the common era to the sophisticated, increasingly more accurate, and therefore more 'truthful' scientific knowledge of cellular physiology, soft tissue biomechanics, and psychobiology (American College of Sports Medicine 1994; McArdle, Katch, and Katch 1996). It is a practically and politically motivated cluster of sciences. Making explicit the political intentions of the exercise sciences in general and the ACSM in particular, George Brooks (1994), in an invited lecture entitled 'Forty

Years of Progress,' celebrating the college's fortieth anniversary, said: 'ACSM through its committees, programs, organizations, and publications has helped *mightily to institutionalize* exercise in the prevention, diagnosis, and treatment of cardiac and other degenerative diseases such as diabetes and obesity. In the past the scientific output in basic and applied exercise physiology has influenced the practice of medicine. Perhaps in the future, exercise physiology will, through ACSM, promote changes in health care delivery at the national level' (36, emphasis added).

The exercise sciences, like virtually all modern sciences, are not simply the detached musings of scholars who see their work as just one among many ways of conceptualizing the human condition. It is a form of knowledge production that is deliberately attempting to change the human condition so that the world will conform to the paradigms of the science. As Bazerman points out, it is a competitive enterprise (Bazerman 1988). Brooks makes this clear in his anniversary lecture. This endeavour is competitive not only at the level of competing concepts, but also at the level of competing professional interests – in the case of the ACSM, of exercise scientists and sports physicians attempting to gain greater control over the health care industry by leveraging national policy on health care, which operates powerful institutional controls on the conduct of human life and health. The exercise sciences are in the most fundamental way engaged in trying to change the reality of the body, to make it function more productively and efficiently. It is the applicability of the exercise sciences, their power to inform human practice, that makes them meaningful and keeps them funded.

The discourse of the applied exercise sciences is academically grounded in the basic sciences of physiology, Newtonian physics, and psychology. Discrete textual fields in the exercise sciences typically fall into the basic disciplinary categories of exercise physiology, biomechanics, and the psychology of exercise and sport. The applied exercise sciences consist of texts on fitness appraisal, exercise prescription, sports training, nutrition, environmental exercise physiology, ergogenic aids for physical and mental performance, and psychology. Because injury is common to sport and physical fitness regimens, there is also a substantial production of scientific texts on the medical treatment of injuries caused by exercise. The applied exercise sciences have a greater tendency than the basic sciences to be multi-disciplinary in their approach. For instance, a standard scientific text on swimming will include research on the physiology, biomechanics, and psychology of competitive swimming, as well as testing for athlete selection, scientifically studied training techniques, nutrition, and management of injuries (Costill, Maglischo, and Richardson 1992).

The multi-disciplinary impulse in exercise science does not extend beyond the physical sciences and the uncritical psychological approaches of behavioural, functionalist, and physiological psychiatry. The critical research of the sociology, anthropology, and history of sport and exercise that I noted briefly in chapter 1 has virtually no presence in the exercise sciences. For example: the *Proceedings* of the Second International Consensus Symposium on Physical Activity, Fitness and Health (Bouchard, Shephard, and Stephens 1992) – a 1,055-page book that purports to review all germane literature on physical activity, fitness, and health – makes no mention of the critical literature. That literature is also completely absent from any of the published lectures from the ACSM's fortieth anniversary. Nor can I find mention of that literature in any scientific manuals on coaching, on exercise testing and prescription, or on fitness instruction.

First, exercise physiology reproduces the concepts of the body used to produce knowledge in basic physiology, which conceptualizes the body as an organism whose processes the linguistic conventions of natural science can accurately represent, whose functions are subject to immutable laws of nature and governed by rules of cause and effect, and whose mechanisms the conventions of reason established in Europe's so-called Enlightenment allow us to know transparently. Exercise physiology understands the body to be an object not unlike any other object, formed by particular operations of chemicals, all of which have molecular and atomic structures that govern their operations. The body is measurable. Measurement is essential to physiology's concept of the body; virtually all the knowledge and power of exercise physiology are the product of measuring the body. Exercise physiology assigns values to and calculates the efficacy of – for example – metabolism, energy expenditure, oxygen uptake, lung volume and capacity, gas exchange and transport, cardiac output, the chemistry of muscle contraction, hormone secretion, and body composition. Exercise physiology measures the effects of exercise on the body's processes. It is driven by the practical quest to control physiological processes in order to increase their efficiency by the optimal organization of the body's energy through diet and physical training of various physiological systems. Instrumental rationality is its guiding principle: how can human reason make the body perform maximally, within particular systematic objectives?

Applied exercise physiology produces texts on the effects of particular training, dietary, and drug regimens on specific practical objectives for improved performance and functional fitness. Many texts present the body's movement in terms of the effects that exercise can have on the 'function of the heart' and on the 'reduction of the risk of cardiovascular illness'; there are many debates between those texts on the kinds, intensities, and quantities of exercise most likely to 'lower the risk of heart disease' (called 'primary prevention') and to 'retard or even stop the development of diagnosed coronary atherosclerosis' (called secondary prevention). Some texts conceive of the body in terms of the effects of exercise on the risk of stroke, hypertension, obesity, diabetes, osteoporosis, cancer, and all-cause mortality, as well as longevity. There are texts on the physiology of many different sports: the sports that have received the most attention are distance running, swimming, cycling, and wrestling. Sport-specific physiology deals with the physiological demands that particular sports make and the development of training and dietary strategies for maximizing the particular physiological capacities that are most relevant to the sport. The texts prescribe very different types of diet, supplements, and training for long-distance running compared to sprinting, for instance. There are texts on the effects of various drugs on sport training and performance, including amphetamines, caffeine, bicarbonate, anabolic steroids, growth hormones, pangamic acid (vitamin B15), creatine, and analgesics.

Second, biomechanics research on exercise and physical fitness produces texts that conceptualize the body as essentially mechanical. It is academically founded in the basic descriptive science of anatomy and in Newtonian physics. Like exercise physiology, biomechanics is preoccupied with measurement and assigns values to the body as mass, force, momentum, weight, impact, pressure, work, power, energy, and so on. Using these measurements, biomechanics calculates the most efficient forms of movement (Hay and Reid 1982). Biomechanical texts have shaped the development of exercise equipment: bicycles, treadmills, weight machines, running shoes, skis, golf clubs, racquets, helmets, balls, and so on. There are texts for different physical activities that analyse movement and suggest the most efficient ways for the body to move for optimal sports performance or for least risk of injury (Nelson 1994). Injury is a major focus of biomechanical texts, both in describing how particular forms of movement contribute to injury, and therefore how to avoid them, and, more prevalent, in prescribing therapies for repairing injuries (Allman 1994).

Third, exercise and sport psychology produces texts that conceptualize mental dimensions of the body. Like the other exercise sciences, its intellectual roots lie in its cognate discipline – in this case, psychology. Unlike physiology, anatomy, and Newtonian physics, however, psychology is theoretically very diverse. While there is no theoretical consensus, some schools are more dominant than others. Unfortunately, there is not space here to review the vast spectrum of theories and approaches and their relative hegemonic positions. Yet despite the considerable differences within psychology, many of the differing approaches of exercise and sport psychology do converge in ways that are germane to my analysis of the technology of physical fitness. Because this branch of psychology aspires to the epistemological and political status of the physical sciences, where measurement is essential, production of quantitative knowledge predominates. Texts attempt to conceptualize, measure, and change the mental (i.e., emotional, intellectual, and behavioural) aspects of life that can detract from athletic performance or 'mental health.'

Mental health, at least in modernized North America, is understood primarily in terms of the *Diagnostic and Statistical Manual*(s) of the American Psychological Association, which offer a taxonomy of that (politically powerful) organization's concepts of the categories of the normal and pathological psyche. In *sport* psychology, there are texts that construct human being under the rubrics of: 'skill acquisition,' 'the role of personality types on athletic performance,' 'the effects of competitiveness, anxiety and aggression on performance,' 'the psychology of motivation,' 'the social psychology of participation in team and individual sports,' 'the effects of age difference on the psychology of sport performance,' and 'the prediction of success and talent identification by psychological profiles.' There are also texts that conceptualize competitive sport, and exercise more generally, in terms of 'exercise adherence,' 'goal setting,' 'self regulation strategies,' 'attention control,' 'optimizing arousal,' 'coping with injuries, overtraining and staleness' (i.e., the experience of no longer finding training interesting and of one's performance therefore not improving). There are texts that purport to measure the effect of exercise on 'mental illnesses,' such as depression, anxiety and personality 'disorders,' as well as on mood, drug use, and 'self-concept,' 'self-esteem,' and 'self-efficacy.'

As in most of the modern sciences, the exercise sciences produce most of their written texts through academic peer-reviewed publishing, with the most prestigious texts published under the governance of scientific societies that restrict membership to individuals who have earned their credentials by working within the established paradigms of their respective sciences, such as the American College of Sports Medicine, the American Medical Association, the American Physiology Association, the American Physiology Society, the International Society for Biomechanics, and the International Society of Sports Psychology. Each of these organizations publishes journals that have names closely resembling those of the society.

As I argued in chapter 1, the exclusivity of such knowledge-governing organizations and the demand that members work within the epistemological paradigms of the scientific discipline in order to publish are crucial for the production of hegemonic knowledge in the field. The authority of the texts of exercise science derives from the strictly controlled cultures of consensus in the various societies regarding the fundamental paradigms that structure thinking about the body. Scientific societies are the custodians and police of their cultures of consensus, enforcing adherence to modern scientific doctrines of the body. In this way they are not unlike the Roman Catholic church's Congregation for the Doctrine of the Faith, whose function is to enforce orthodoxy in the church. This is not to say that their control is total; within the fundamental doctrine of the body to which the exercise sciences adhere there is considerable debate – what quantities and intensities of exercise produce the most effective results, what dietary supplements are most effective and in what quantity and what combinations, what the ideal ratio is of fat to lean, and so on. But the fundamental epistemological paradigms for producing knowledge in their journals establish a limiting parergonal logic for them – a logic that I attempt to reveal in my deconstruction in chapter 4.

The texts of the academic exercise sciences are inscribed outside the research laboratory and the world of academic publishing. The Canadian Society for Exercise Physiology (CSEP), for instance, runs a national program for appraising physical fitness and prescribing exercise. Through its National Fitness Appraisal Certification and Accreditation Program, the CSEP credentiallizes fitness appraisers and publishes newsletters telling them about recent developments in the field. Similarly, in the United States, the American College of Sports Medicine (ACSM) oversees accreditation in physical fitness testing and exercise prescription, reproducing a variety of texts that are intended to disseminate its positions on exercise and practice based on scientific research, including its *Resource Guidelines for Exercise Testing and Prescription* (1993). Testing of physical fitness and prescribing exercise are widespread practised in community and university athletic facilities, for both competitive athletes and the general population. Most commercial fitness clubs offer, indeed encourage, both practices. In Australia and the United Kingdom, professional organizations – the Australian Association for Exercise and Sport Science and the British Association of Sport and Exercise Science, respectively – maintain registers of accredited fitness testers and exercise and 'lifestyle consultants.'

While testing and prescription are not subject to government legislation in the same way as medical diagnosis and the prescription of pharmaceutical products, organizations such as the CSEP and the ACSM are trying to promote the professional monopolies of their accredited appraisers, thus further insinuating the conceptual universe of the exercise sciences into the daily practice of life (Rouse 1987, 226ff).

The doctrine of the body and health common to the exercise sciences is also promulgated through higher education. Most prospective teachers of physical education in schools, and many workers in the fitness industry, study in university or college programs, where they learn the exercise sciences. There are consequently many standard textbooks on the discipline. Typically, programs are dominated by the positivist physical and psychological exercise sciences, and many of the departments are now called 'kinesiology' – a scientific-sounding word that is used to give greater credibility to physical education. So the typical program emphasizes the academic study of anatomy, basic physiology, exercise physiology, environmental physiology, sport medicine, biomechanics, motor learning, exercise prescription, adapted and corrective exercise, cellular physiology, nutrition, sport psychology, psycho-social development, quantitative research design and statistics, administrative theory and practice, epidemiology, and the psychophysiology of stress. In this emphasis they resemble other health sciences (medicine, dentistry, pharmacy, nursing, physiotherapy, and so on).[3] Most schools offer one or two courses in the history or sociology of physical education, and a few, other socio-cultural options. But such courses are usually ancillary to the core curriculum (Demers 1988; Harvey 1986; Kirk 1986; 1994; MacIntosh 1986; MacIntosh and Whitson 1990; McKay, Gore, and Kirk 1990).

Popular Texts

The exercise sciences also reproduce their doctrines in a plethora of popular exercise books, magazines, web sites, and videos. These texts reproduce, to varying degrees, the knowledge that is produced in the exercise sciences. Their power comes from their consumer appeal, market orientation, practicality, and immediate applicability to the everyday lives of their target consumers. They are positioned explicitly in the logics of consumer culture: they construct or highlight a personal lack in the consumer's life and suggest a pattern of consumption that promises to fill that gap. Depending on the particular popular text, it will draw more or less rigorously on the epistemic authority and actual technological power of the exercise sciences to deliver their consumer promise. Some are exacting in their application of the exercise sciences, and others might be called 'quackery' by exercise scientists. There are several market niches for these texts, such as:

- **rehabilitation**: for example, *The Sports Medicine Bible: Prevent, Detect, and Treat Your Sports Injures through the Latest Medical Techniques* (Micheli and Jenkins 1995)
- **healthy living**: for example, *Athletic Forever: The Kerlen–Jobe Orthopaedic Clinic Plan for Lifetime Fitness* (Jobe, ElAttrache, and Rand 1999)
- **body shaping**: for example, *The Complete Book of Butt and Legs: Over One Hundred Exercises [and] Dozens of Routines for home and Gym. Get the Best Results in the Shortest Time* (Brungardt, Brungardt, and Brungardt 1995)
- **recreational sport performance**: for example, *The Triathlete's Training Bible: A Complete Training Guide for the Competitive Multisport Athlete* (Friel 1998)
- **personal motivation**: for example, *Get Motivated: Daily Psych-Ups* (Farley and Curry 1994).

There is considerable market cross-over between these books.

In the ensemble of popular texts on the technology of physical fitness, commercial interests are more obvious than in the academic texts of journals, manuals, and college textbooks outlined above. Take, for example, *Fitness for Dummies*™ (Schlosberg and Neporent 1996), part of two series of 'Dummies' and 'Idiots' books that started as computer guides for people who knew little about computers. Their market has expanded well beyond computers; there are thirteen titles in the 'Dummies' series alone on how to become fit, healthy, athletic, beautiful. The books include advertisements for equipment and services and devote considerable space to advice on consuming fitness and other related products, as well as addresses for contacting manufactures of equipment and services. Nevertheless, *Fitness for Dummies*™ calls significantly on all three of the academic exercise sciences for the training programs that it recommends. While one of the authors is a fitness journalist, the other (Liz Neporent) has a graduate degree in exercise physiology and 'is certified by the American Council on Exercise, the American College of Sports Medicine and the National Strength and Conditioning Association' (Schlosberg and Neporent 1996, xxii). Certainly not all the popular texts are rigorous in their application of the exercise sciences. Many of the fitness magazines, for instance, tend to promote programs of immoderate weight reduction, through crash diets and intense exercise, which the health-oriented exercise sciences argue is dangerously unhealthy. Magazines and videos are highly visual media, and the bodies portrayed in them are almost invariably extraordinarily lean. Most of the space in the magazines goes to display advertisements, many of which claim 'scientific proof' for their products' effectiveness, even when the claims are clearly at odds with current consensus in the exercise sciences. For example, there are often ads for exercise machines that claim to reduce fat specifically around the waist. But the texts of exercise physiology claim that 'spot lipid reduction' is not possible, since fats are metabolized systemically rather than locally.

While their use of exercise science can be selective and is often driven by an obvious profit motive, popular texts do reproduce remarkably well the fundamental *technological* doctrines of the body that are essential to the exercise sciences. This I attempt to show below in the deconstruction of the intertextual ensemble. There are two more textual fields in the intertextual ensemble of the technology of physical fitness that need to be outlined.

Physical Fitness Products

The technology of physical fitness circulates in a consumer economy of goods and services. Services include membership in fitness and sports clubs and centres, which offer fitness appraisal and exercise prescription, exercise equipment and space, instruction, personal trainers, various aerobic exercise classes, massage, change rooms, showers, saunas, as well as goods. Goods include exercise equipment, clothing, special foods, dietary supplements, therapeutic technologies, cosmetics, and body monitoring equipment such as weigh-scales, heart monitors, and fat callipers.

Physical fitness facilities produce a cornucopia of texts on the body. Fitness appraisal and exercise prescription, for instance, are staples of fitness centres; the more commercial operations give staff members an opportunity to appraise the body of a client by testing and writing texts about them and then recommending fitness products that the company sells. Typically, when a person joins a commercial fitness facility, he or she will be encouraged to undergo a fitness appraisal that will produce texts on his or her body specifically, as well as an individualized prescription to fill the body's lacks. The facility will also urge retesting in order to monitor the body's changes, or lack thereof, and prescribe alternative practices and patterns of fitness product consumption.

The Canadian Physical Activity Fitness and Lifestyle Assessment (CPAFLA) does an appraisal of fitness that is widespread in Canada and is similar to scientific tests used in other countries. In a fitness appraisal, the body is measured, measurements are recorded, calculations are made, an assessment is given, and a way of life is prescribed. Most appraisals consist of anthropometric measurements of height, weight, skinfold thickness, resting heart rate and blood pressure, aerobic capacity, hand strength, and upper-, middle-, and lower-body strength. Sometimes an electrocardiogram is taken, clients receive computer printouts of the results. They contribute to this narrative on their own bodies not only by performing the tasks recorded by the appraiser, but also by writing responses to questionnaires about their way of life, as well as by participating in an ongoing confessional dialogue with the appraiser throughout the assessment.

The appraiser uses the information from the questionnaire and discussions to convince the client to change his or her way of life, pointing out aspects of the participant's life that lend themselves to increased physical activity and to leading a different life. For example, one manual suggests the following: 'I see that you like going for a walk once a day. You might want to start walking twice a day. Have you ever thought of jogging? You might like that too' (Canadian Association of Sport Sciences 1987a). Even if the participant is found to be extremely fit, the appraiser will suggest strategies for improvement: 'Your VO_2 of 31mL/Kg/min is at the 90 percentile. You are obviously a seasoned exerciser and you are congratulated on your progress. For you to maintain your score be sure to continue with the same volume of work. If you wish to further your score it will be necessary for you to become involved with some more advanced training such as aerobic intervals which increase intensity while still allow [sic] a long duration workout. Consult a training specialist for this kind of program' (from a computer printout of the results of a fitness appraisal done at the University of Toronto).

Fitness appraisal is explicitly grounded in the three exercise sciences: exercise physiology, biomechanics, and exercise psychology. The stated purpose of fitness testing is to change people's behaviour. The Canadian test was developed to be a 'springboard for lifestyle change' – indeed, 'the most important aspect of the ... appraisal process is the promotion of a physically active, wellness-oriented lifestyle' (Canadian Association of Sport Sciences 1987a, 7). So while physiology and biomechanics are the core of the appraisal, for its application to the general public the most recent version of the appraisal (Canadian Society for Exercise Physiology 1996) stresses the motivational psychology of exercise, using the physiological and biomechanical texts that it produces as part of the motivational strategy. Physical fitness appraisal, reproducing the knowledge-power that is produced in the exercise sciences, produces texts on individual lives. The purpose of those individualized texts is to extend the doctrinal worldview of the exercise sciences out from the laboratory and the world of academic publishing and into the everyday lives of the population.

In addition to physical fitness appraisal, fitness facilities produce a plethora of texts on the body. For instance, commercial clubs oriented to body sculpting often display pictures of buff and lean fitness practitioners, presumably to inspire the clients to produce their own bodies similarly. These clubs frequently have a policy of hiring only those employees whose bodies exemplify the sculpted look. Personal trainers work with customers to fine-tune the exercise prescription on a daily basis and to motivate the customer to produce results. Wealthy clients will sometimes even take their trainers with them when they travel. The role of the personal trainer in the intertextual ensemble is to produce texts on the client's body at every workout. These texts are sometimes written in a log book; but they are frequently verbal, as the trainer describes the body and progress to the client, and they are also physical, as the trainer exemplifies with his or her body how the client's body should be, as well as aiding in the actual conduct of the exercise.

At most facilities, exercise machines have pictures that portray how the body is to be inserted into the machines, as well as written texts on how to use them. The machines are calibrated so that the user can set its functions to a selected intensity. Computerized aerobic training machines such as stair climbers, treadmills, stationary bicycles, and rowing ergometers invite the user to key in his or her age, weight, and preference for style and length of workout, and they will program a workout of varying intensities, inform the user when he or she is not working hard enough, record the number of calories being burned, and so on. Some machines, by monitoring the heart rate, automatically adjust the resistance up or down in order to force the exerciser's heart to remain in the training zone that has been programmed. For instance, the Cateye EC-1600 stationary bicycle is advertised as offering the following: 'Tri-level fitness test plus 5 training programs: Automatic Training, Isopower Training, Interval Training, Hill Profile Training and Manual Training. Photo-optic earlobe sensor for extremely accurate heart rate readings, patented data card system for one button start-up. 7 continuously monitored biofeedback functions plus read-outs of 25 mechanical and physiological factors. Printouts of 5 key biofeedback functions every 30 seconds – for daily, weekly, and monthly comparisons. Emergency shut off system at upper heart-rate limit. Patented electromagnetic resistance system with additional fly-wheel for smooth, natural pedal movement (http://www.bodytrends. com/products/bike/cateye1600.htm).'

Adhering closely to the laboratory paradigms of exercise science, technological approaches to physical fitness measure the protocols and effects of exercise. The act of measuring is itself a textual production, albeit fleeting and dependent on memory. For instance, one can weigh oneself on a weekly basis and keep in mind the fluctuations in weight, thus producing and preserving a memory text of the body in the *logos* of weight measurement. Similarly, one can swim a particular number of laps several times a week, or do a weight-lifting routine, counting the number of repetitions, sets, and weight of each exercise, remember what one did the last time, and adjust the different elements the next time accordingly, thus producing and preserving memory texts of the body in the hermeneutical traditions of lap swimming and weight lifting. These measurements contextualize important aspects of the meaning of the moving body in terms of stasis or progress in intensity and duration of exercises, for instance. These measurements construct an interpretive framework.[4] Such casual remembering of measurements does not offer the 'resolution,' to borrow Foucault's photographic metaphor, that inscription has. There are therefore technologies for inscribing measurements. Keeping a log book is one such technique, but it is highly dependent on the subjectivity of the recorder, be it the exerciser or a coach/trainer. The stationary bicycle described above prints out results so that the exerciser can calculate his or her development over time. A dedicated exerciser would subsequently inscribe these scientifically objective results in a log book.

As both Rouse and Bazerman suggest, the value of science comes from the fact that 'it works,' and it does so because the laboratory is able to produce reality by controlling the events of an experiment. What is revealed in a (successful) laboratory experiment is the reality that will come to presence when something is marshalled to presence in accordance with the paradigms and objectives of the experiment. For this to take place, events must strictly adhere to a protocol, and the results must be accurately and objectively reported. Otherwise there is no sure way of knowing what the experiment produced. In exercise science, adherence to protocol is accomplished by ensuring that the body makes itself present in the service of the experiment by fitting the machinery of the experiment and by performing in ways that can be measured objectively. I recall one of my physiology colleagues giving a lecture on his research in which he demonstrated, with slides, how he performed an experiment in which he had tied a live rat to a peg, isolated its gastrocnemius muscle, and inserted electrodes that compelled the muscle to twitch at the command of a computer program that he had designed. Another computer recorded the results. The angles of the rat's leg were carefully measured to ensure that it fitted the machine in accordance with the protocol. Electrical stimulation compelled the rat to perform according to the requirements of the experiment. The rat's performance was then measured, following which the rat was 'sacrificed.'

Humans are used in similar experiments, although not usually so invasively. The controlled and isolated use of rats and humans is common experimental practice in exercise physiology, biomechanics, and psychology. In biomechanics subjects are strapped into machines and psychologically urged to perform a task strictly within the demands of the protocol. A ubiquitous photo illustration in exercise physiology texts shows a person running on a treadmill with a gas collector strapped to his mouth, a tube leading to a Beckman metabolic cart, electro-cardiographic electrodes attached to various parts of his body, a blood pressure cuff on his arm, a computer wired to the data-gathering equipment, and scientists monitoring the procedure. In the fitness appraisal of CPAFLA, subjects exercise to the strictly determined temporal beat of music. The music ensures the machine–body fit, which in turn makes it possible to measure the performance more or less accurately. In science, objective, electro-mechanically produced, measurable data are considered more accurate than the subjective experience of the exerciser. Similarly, in the everyday practice of exercise, efficiency and accuracy are best served when the exerciser conforms most strictly to a scientific protocol, rather than according to his or her free desire. That is most effectively accomplished when the movement and exertion are fully subject to controlled conditions.

Exercise science 'works' because it can coerce reality into appearing in ways that are coherent with its various projects, and it does so through procedures of control, measurement, and adjustment. One of the ways whereby the precision and control of the research lab reach into everyday life is through commercially available equipment such as monitors of heart rate, which attempt to configure and control the desire of exercises such that they resist the temptation to pay attention to how they feel and exercise instead according to the objective data and predetermined protocol that has been programmed into the mini-computer on their wrist. The 'Vantage NV' heart rate monitor, for example, can be programmed to target heart rate zones; whenever the exerciser's pulse goes above or below the targeted heart rate, an alarm sounds, signalling that the exerciser should bring the rate back into the targeted zone. (Different kinds of training are more physiologically effective at different intensities; the heart rate codes the intensity.) So that the exerciser can determine his or her effectiveness in adhering to the exercise protocol over the duration of the workout, the monitor will compute the time spent above and below the targeted zone, as well as the average rate for the entire workout. One approach to scientific training entails apportioning exercise intensity over various distances – it is called splitting, the point being to rationalize energy expenditure (desire) so that one does not go too fast or too slow during different parts of the bout in order that one will by the end have maximized efficient expenditure of energy. The 'Vantage NV' therefore records split times with their corresponding heart rates; this codes for the exerciser the objective speed and intensity at different intervals over time. Because the speed of heart rate recovery after exercise (how quickly the heart rate returns to its pre-exercise rate) is an indicator of an overall physiological efficiency, the monitor also calculates and records recovery rates through the workout. Rather than recording all this data in a handwritten log book, one can download the data to a larger computer and to programs that can then use the data to calculate more efficient, individualized training protocols for the future.

Popular Representations of the Fit Body

The display of the living, active, fit body itself constitutes a textual field. While the display of the fit body is not new – it was a feature of the gymnasium (Latin, from Greek *gumnasion*: from *gumnazo*, exercise, from *gumnos*, naked) of classical Greece – its commodification and mass production as a technological artefact of consumer culture are. In Charles Atlas's famous advertisements in men's magazines in the postwar era, it was at the beach where the partially clad skinny young man had sand kicked in his face by the big, fit, muscular brute, who 'stole' his girlfriend. Beaches have continued to be important sites for the display of the sculpted body. But popular spaces for such display have expanded considerably in many parts of the world over the last two decades: 'casually' in city parks, on city streets, in dance clubs, bars, and baths, and 'deliberately,' where such bodies are produced in fitness centres, at swimming pools, and at athletic events, where increasingly smaller lycra sports clothes reveal more and more of the body's contours.[5]

We can also read such actual bodies-on-display in the intertextuality of media representations of the body. In that textual field, representations of the body by the fashion industry occupy considerable visual semiotic space, circumscribing popular visions of the body-beautiful with images of the tight, technologically produced, fit body. On billboards, on public transit, in magazines, in movies, and on television, the sculpted body is ubiquitous in advertisements for underwear, jeans, cologne, casual wear, sports gear, high-energy foods, and so on. The very buff Marky Mark, for instance was featured in a high-profile

Calvin Klein underwear campaign. Exemplifying the crossing of fields of the intertextual ensemble of physical fitness, as I mentioned above, Marky Mark also markets an exercise video that demonstrates not only his technologically produced body, but also a series of standard exercises and advice on diet, based on scientific research on muscle hypertrophy and control of adiposity, as well as on long-standing practices in body building.

The omnipresence of these popular representations of the fit body undoubtedly contextualize the ways in which people read bodies, whether they themselves follow exercise and dietary regimens or not. It is a powerful context. Foucault points out that where there is power there is resistance. Explicit, albeit minority, nodes of resistance have emerged in the media and in popular culture. British television cooking show celebrities the 'Two Fat Ladies' – the recently deceased Jennifer Paterson and Clarissa Dickson Wright – and Rosie O'Donnell, who stars in a popular U.S. television talk show, champion themselves and their corpulent bodies as alternatives to the hegemony of the technologically fit body. In gay male culture, the minority 'bear culture' features large, but not buff, hirsute men.

The display of the 'desirable,' fit body is a major element in the film and television industry, which, like advertising, helps contextualize popular cultural imagery. While a comprehensive discussion of such use there of the fit, sculpted body is beyond the scope of this book, I wish to mention a few of the many names that have led the phenomenon: Cher, Cindy Crawford, Jane Fonda, Christopher Reeves, Arnold Schwarzenegger, and Sylvester Stallone, for example. At the time of writing, one of the most popular American television 'dramas' in the entire world is 'Baywatch,' a weekly program ostensibly about lifeguarding on a California beach. It deals directly with the consumption of the desirability of physically fit, active bodies, carefully sculpted according to the different hegemonic expectations of masculine and feminine genders, as exemplified by David Charet, David Chokachi, Nicole Eggert, David Hasselhoff, and Pamela Lee. This program makes explicit links between the bodies of the stars and the audience: in conjunction with the large North American fitness club chain Bally's, the television program sponsors a series of triathlons across the United States, some of which include actors from the show, and the promotions for which all include photos of sculpted competitors and models. The website offers training advice and multiple links for sculpting the body.

Conclusion: The Intertextual Ensemble

People can read the *ensemble* of texts of physical fitness in multiple and highly fragmented ways. No one, of course, will have looked at the entire ensemble, and few will have read in all the fields. For instance, one reader may have seen some 'infomercials' about exercise videos on television, had a fitness appraisal, and received instruction from a personal trainer on weight training, never having seen any of the academic texts on fitness. Another concerned about his health, having been advised by his physician to exercise and being aware of the role of exercise in government guidelines on health promotion, may read only *Fitness for Dummies*™. Or one could be a graduate of a master of science program in kinesiology, having therefore been an avid reader of the natural science journals and textbooks in exercise physiology and perhaps also be a dedicated recreational soccer player and coach, yet she may not have read much of anything in the popular literature, except perhaps a soccer magazine; but like most people she would have seen the lean, buff bodies that are ubiquitous in the popular media.

The textual ensemble operates as an ensemble not because there are omniscient readers 'who have seen it all,' but operated out of the partial and differing perspectives that develop as a result of the multifaceted and multimediated reproduction of the ensemble. I now argue that while each textual field and indeed different texts within each field represent the technology of physical fitness in somewhat different ways, throughout the ensemble there is a common, essential (in Heidegger's sense) reading and writing of the body, of its future, and of its place in the political and ecological scheme of things. This is so, despite departures from such a reading in a sizeable minority of texts, including some that I mentioned above in the Introduction. And just as multiplicity and fragmentation occur within the intertextual ensemble, so too they exist among its readers and subjects. These texts emanate from and speak mostly to the middle- and upper-class readers of (post)modern global popular and techno-scientific culture. And individuals informed by the ensemble are not simply passive recipients of its philosophy of life. The reproduction of texts in life is a many-layered enterprise. While the ensemble writes a way of life that I argue is profoundly nihilistic, it is not always successful in its project.

Luce Irigaray (cited by Grosz 1995, 84) claims that the 'specificity of the female morphology and its independence from and resistance to the penetration of masculine scrutiny' (which is arguably what the intertextual ensemble of the technology of physical fitness largely is) leaves women space that is free of some discourses, albeit a restricted kind of freedom. There is a valuable insight here: there are regions of desire, of the body, dimensions of being human, of being at all, that may be inaccessible to discourses – particularly nihilistic ones – and they are inaccessible precisely because of the violence of the discourses. There may be dimensions of being that cannot be violated. Incomprehensible to the violent, parergonal logic of modern technology, such dimensions are rendered second, ignored but not eradicated. Such regions are culturally enframed in such a way that they may be more accessible to those who are made second/other than to those who fit the culture.

This is one of the crucial discoveries of postcolonial studies: even when violently colonized, elements of the indigenous can remain, albeit recast, despite the coloniz(ed) experience (Spivak 1995). Similarly, with the body that is represented in the texts of the technology of physical fitness: there may be something of the indigenous, subaltern dimensions of the body that remains, even for the most avid disciple of the technology. I leave it to the readers of this book to reflect on the extent to which the project of the technology of physical fitness is reproduced in their own lives, in those whom they know, and in the institutions and cultures to which they are exposed. Indeed, the enduring hope of my analysis is that there be *many* ways in which technology has not been successful and that there are therefore real possibilities for resisting or even transcending the modern technological project, both individually and collectively. My interrogation of the texts of the technology of physical fitness is not a judgment on the lived production of desire for those who 'read' and live within the ensemble. It is instead an interrogation of the *direction* that the texts chart for desire: do they attempt to map an *identity* with pouvoir, or do they seek to open a compassionate (empty) space for becoming *different*?

Each field, and different texts within each field, code the body in different ways: The texts of exercise science obviously work within the conventions of modern scientific writing. They are mostly reviewed by peers. Except for a relatively unnoticed area of qualitative psychology, they all engage in measurement and operate under the assumption that the numbers and calculations that they use in their research correspond to human realities – i.e., that there is an accurate correlation between the texts' signifying practices and the bodies that they attempt to signify. They all purport to be objective representations of the functions of exercise, independent of motives other than the pursuit of truth.

But within each of the sciences there are many different systems of codification, depending on what parameters are being measured. Within exercise physiology, for example, various areas of research reproduce quite different coding systems – for example, whole-body exercise physiology, with its concern for macro-systemic codes for aerobic capacity, such as VO_2max., measured in millilitres of oxygen per kilogram of body weight per minute, versus cellular physiology, with its microsystemic codes for cardiac concentrations of lactate, glycogen, or glucose, measured in millimoles per milligram of tissue. And obviously government policies, scientific texts, popular texts, the products of physical fitness, and different displays of the fit body call on a variety of coding systems and contexts that have their points of both difference and convergence. Some are more scientifically rigorous than others, some have less clear commercial impetus than others, and some are more open to human differences (for example, the almost-pervasive reproduction of the cult of extreme slenderness in the popular texts, versus the advocacy of a spectrum of body shapes and adiposity in government and health science texts).

But all these differences are superficial. For virtually all the texts and textual fields outlined above reproduce basic doctrines of the body and how desire should unfold. What they share in common is important. Indeed, exploring that commonality is key to appreciating the problems of the technology of physical fitness. The intertextual ensemble coheres in its basic conceptualization of and engagement with the body, which it does within the dominant mythology of the body in modernity. That fundamental coherence knits together the different fields of the ensemble, so that while a reader is probably exposed to only parts of the whole, he or she may still be comprehensively indoctrinated into the fundamental *logos* of the body that those texts represent. All these texts describe, inscribe, and prescribe a narrative of the body that is made intelligible and legitimate by reference to a mythology of the body grounded in a plan for salvation (a soteriology) both individual and collective. Appealing to the philosophy of the limit, I next draw out of this intertextual ensemble the underlying doctrine of human life that gives the technology of physical fitness its intelligibility and apparent legitimacy.

Pouvoir, as I said in chapter 2, develops the puissance of desire as a resource. The intertextual ensemble writes the program for this resource development and management through government and nongovernment policies on health and fitness, scientific research, fitness appraisal, exercise and dietary regimens, and popular representations of the fit body. It does so by inscribing a system for becoming human, attempting to form the parameters of what Toby Miller has called the 'well-tempered self,' which I suggest is the properly managed modern technological subject. This is the subject recounted in Foucault's theory of 'subjection' – i.e., it is about the ways in which 'people are invited or incited to recognize their moral obligations' (cited in Miller 1993, xiii). This is a subject that is formed essentially in the parergonal logic of domination that runs the Western cultural construction of being – bell hooks (1994) has said that we live in a 'culture of domination' and that we are so deeply embedded in it that it has become virtually impossible for us to imagine any other organization of moral life; we are the subjects of domination. The intertextual ensemble writes the story of a particular kind of subject formation, a configuration that I attempt to show in the next chapter is anthropocentric, egocentric, phallocentric, and technocentric – in short, the modern Western subject. Our deconstructive task therefore is to see how that system attempts to construct a parergonal logic for puissance. Where do these texts attempt to take their readers? Where do they fail to take the readers? What is left out of this system?

4

Writing the Fascist Body:
Description, Inscription, Prescription

When the man lies down on the Bed and it begins to vibrate, the Harrow is lowered onto his body. It regulates itself automatically so that the needles barely touch his skin; once contact is made the steel ribbon stiffens immediately into a rigid band ... As it quivers, its points pierce the skin of the body which is itself quivering from the vibration of the bed ... There are two kinds of needles arranged in multiple patterns. Each long needle has a short one beside it. The long needle does the writing, and the short needle sprays a jet of water to wash away the blood and keep the inscription clear ... The Harrow is beginning to write; when it finishes the first draft of the inscription on the back, the layer of cotton-wool begins to roll and slowly turns the body over, to give the Harrow fresh space for writing. Meanwhile the raw part that has been written on lies on the cotton-wool, which is specially prepared to staunch the bleeding and so makes ready for a new deepening of the script ... So it keeps on writing deeper and deeper ... The man begins to understand the inscription, he purses his mouth as if he was listening. You have seen how difficult it was to decipher the script with one's eyes; but our man deciphers it with his wounds.

Franz Kafka 1961, 176–80

The intertextual ensemble reviewed in the previous chapter *calls* the body. Exercise physiology, for instance, calls the body 'functionally organic.' Biomechanics calls the body 'mechanical.' Exercise psychology calls desire 'normal' or 'abnormal.' The popular cult of slimness calls the body 'fat,' 'fit,' 'beautiful,' or 'sexy.' Health promotion calls some bodies 'at risk' or 'economically underproductive.' Throughout the intertextual ensemble, the body is called things.

As Heidegger points out, calling means naming. For example, the exercise sciences name the parts and functions of the cardiovascular system – that's how it knows the body. When I called my puppy 'Jascha,' I gave him that name. And now that he is a mature dog, when I call that name, he comes, most of the time. Calling and naming are dynamic events. To call is also to summon, to bring that which is called nearer to the caller (Heidegger 1971, 198). Such nearness is not just a physical proximity, as when I call my dog and he comes over to me. That which is called is brought nearer by virtue of being shown within the conceptual universe (i.e., the parergonal logic) of the caller or calling, as the kind of being that it has been called.

And so, when exercise physiology calls the body a functional organism with a cardiovascular system that can be measured, calculated, and trained to function more efficiently, it summons the body forth **as** what it has been called. The body is summoned to account for itself as a functional organism, and only as such. How and what the body is called has a profound effect on what appears in the various texts of the technology of physical fitness. How does the technology of physical fitness call the body in its essence? How does it make puissance come to presence? How do its texts use their sundry languages, words, pictures, apparatuses, procedures, practices, and institutions to call the body forth, and to what end? What, in short, do they call on the body to become?

For the philosophy of the limit, the technological calling of the body and the words that it uses warrant careful attention, so that we can know what is called and what is not. Calvin Luther Martin (1992) speaks of 'words as sculptors of space, as turn-keys: liberators or jailers of the powers about us' (25). Martin's observation suggests alternatives: our language can liberate (deterritorialize) puissance or confine (reterritorialize) it. The words that we use to script the body in physical fitness have enormous power to liberate or to subjugate. The language of the technology of physical fitness can set the horizons of bodily perception: what do I perceive when I understand the body – that is, understand the puissance of desire – in the language of the texts of physical fitness? David Abram (1983) believes that there is more to perception than simply looking at something, to use the metaphor of sight. Perception, he says, is communication. The words that we use to describe what appears to us, indeed the language that we use in order to perceive at all, calls that which appears to do so as what we have called it. This is an extraordinarily powerful force. And it has a history of some of the most dreadful abuse. The Nazis, for instance, calling the Jews 'filthy vermin,' forced them to appear in the eyes of Nazis as such and to be disposed of as such. As Heidegger writes, to name a thing is to call it into being, as what it is called. Is there listening in such calling? Does the caller hear?

Heidegger said that the *ta mathemata* of science lays over phenomena a conceptual framework, so that that which appears does so within the framework. 'The observer's choice of what he shall look for has an inescapable consequence for what he shall find' (Wheeler 1982, 13). And as Rouse and as Menser and Aronowitz argue, science is not just a theoretical enterprise, but a highly engaged one that uses its technological powers as well as its embeddedness in modern techno-culture to produce realities that are consistent with its epistemic paradigms (Menser and Aronowitz 1996; Rouse 1987). Keep in mind that modern technology makes what is there appear as a resource, both for its local products of academic knowledge and for the larger socio-economic project of managing, developing, and exploiting resources. So when the technology of physical fitness calls the body, it is engaging in a powerful act of *making* the body appear. It is a form of perception that is very one-sided: the only perception that matters, the one that controls how things appear, is the perception that is enframed by what is already known in advance of an encounter with a phenomenon.

Abram comments: 'Perception has to be understood and recognized as reciprocal exchange. When we see things we are also being seen by them. When we hear things we are also being heard. Perception is a type of communication that precedes language' (as cited in Calvin Luther Martin 1992, 24). What does desire hear when called to presence technologically? As we read our bodies in the texts of physical fitness, how much of *puissance's reading* of our act of technological reading and producing do we hear in return? Is there reciprocal communication? Alterity, which is the ethical commitment of the philosophy of the limit, demands that we open our awareness to that which is made other to our reading, naming, and consequent selective summoning into presence of the infinitely possible.

Does the technology of resource management listen to what the sources that have been re-sourced call out? Does the technology of physical fitness listen at all to the source (puissance) that it is resourcing (pouvoir). I suggest that if we are aware of our being perceived by things, we may become more aware of how we are acting on things. This is true not only of paying attention to our relationships with the environment – the ecological field of being that surrounds us and gives us life – but also of paying attention to our 'own' bodies. This means heightening our awareness of how the body perceives the scripting discourses that we are using to understand and produce the body. That is, it is a matter of trying to see the effects that our language – our scripting conventions in the technoculture of physical fitness – have on the body, from the perspective of *the body*. It is a matter of being aware of the body not only as an object of the language of techno-science, but also as a perceptive subject and possible critic of techno-science. But if we keep in mind that there may be a powerful way of perceiving the body and desire – a way that is rendered second in the parergonal logic of the technology of physical fitness – it may help us to appreciate more fully what happens when the body is called by the intertextual ensemble of physical fitness.

The intertextual ensemble forms a *simulacrum* of desire. For Deleuze, the simulacrum is not the ethereal copy for which there is no original, which is Baudriallard's well-known formulation. 'A common definition of the simulacrum is a copy of a copy whose relation to the model has become so attenuated that it can no longer be properly said to be a copy. It stands on its own as a copy without a model. Fredric Jameson cites the example of photorealism. The painting is a copy not of reality but of a photograph which is already a copy of the original' (Massumi 1997, 2). Baudrillard says that the process has gone so far that there is no longer a real referent for signs, but only signs of signs. Deleuze has a much more materialist understanding: the simulacrum is a partial concretization of potential in a form that serves political-ideological ends, which I am arguing in the case of the technology of physical fitness is the reformation of puissance in the pouvoir of modern resource management. 'Simulation does not *replace* reality ... it *appropriates* reality in the operation of a despotic overcoding' (Massumi 1997, 3). By codifying desire, the simulacrum insinuates a reality that replaces desire's puissant capacity to create free connections. The simulacrum, thus understood, abstracts from bodies a 'transcendental plane of ideal identities and then folds that ideal dimension back on to bodies in order to force them to conform to the distribution it lays out for them' (2). It is the simulacrum that the dynamics of desire forms and produces social identities. The simulacrum charts a future for presencing by writing the plane of identity into the space of absence in the drawing-penetrating-absence-presence of movement. It loads the space of movement by charting the distributions of movement's expenditure in accordance with the parergonal logics of ideal identities (be they the expectations of gender, race, class, or the technologically functioning cybernetic organism).

In my discussion of Heidegger's analysis of modern technology in chapter 2 above, I claimed that modern technology enframes and thus marshals beings as resources. It is a profound transformation of the inherent freedom of being in the service of social, cultural, and economic projects. The word 'resource' comes from the Latin root *surgere*, which means to arise. So, when something is re-sourced, it is made to arise or to become present, prosaically in accordance with socio-cultural projects rather than poetically in the mysterious original freedom of Being, of becoming the Body without Organs (BwO). In the technology of physical fitness, the inherent freedom of our BwO, the freedom of puissance, is re-sourced by the pouvoir of this simulacrum. The intertextual ensemble codes desire in order to make it arise in a particular way. The technology of physical fitness simulates desire in a codifying ensemble of texts and practices that extort from the infinity of being a finite picture of and plan for what is possible. It does so by a tripartite process of writing codes for the body: description, inscription and prescription. I begin with a brief overview of each of these and follow with three sections that deconstruct in turn the codes that description, inscription, and prescription represent in the technology of physical fitness.

First, description establishes the overarching logos, the conceptual universe, the cosmology, the hermeneutic circle, the 'particular grammar' (Miller 1993), or what Heidegger calls the 'as structure,' that renders the body comprehensible and thus accessible to the technological mode of making human and other beings manifest. The descriptive process calls the body as technologically intelligible, in such a way that it can be understood and thus organized as a potential resource. Applying Deleuze and Guattari's work suggests that description sketches the technological framework for coding and therefore for territorializing the flow of desire in the abstract terms of value. Drawing on Cornell, we can say that it invokes the parergonal logic for perceiving the body, marking what can and cannot be included in the system for understanding and organizing the body's past, present, and future. And in terms of Barthes: in describing the body, the intertextual ensemble locates the body within the naturalizing myths of modernity, situating the technology of physical fitness in modernity's cosmology of humanity, its dominant place in the totality of the earth, and its never-ending technological struggle to gain that control over life which will ensure the sovereignty of that which exalts itself as lord of both the earth and itself. Without the invocation of that conceptual universe, the notion that the body can be measured, that it can and should be changed by technologies of physical fitness in order to have greater control over its destiny (be it health, longevity, productivity, or desirability), would be meaningless, if not ludicrous.

Second, inscription consists of those textual practices, or what Foucault calls micro-technologies, that insinuate the modern logos, the parergonal logics, the evaluative codes, or the hermeneutics of the technological body into the lives of individual human beings. Inscription is literally the process of writing the technology of physical fitness into individual bodies. Examination and confessional practices inscribe the technology – they compel the body to account for itself in the parergonality of the conceptual universe that the technology describes. A fitness test, for instance, codes the body in the hermeneutics of that technology and measures it for its ability to conform to the myth of the body that the exercise sciences have described. Similarly, evaluating one's own body in comparison with the sleek bodies of advertising, one inscribes the parergonal logics of the buff and slender, technologically produced body of consumer culture onto one's own body. Similar acts of inscription occur when one appreciates (or does not appreciate) the bodies of one's friends and lovers in accordance with fashions of buff and lean, for example.

Third, prescription writes futures of the body and desire within the cosmology, mythology, and soteriology of the technology of physical fitness. Sometimes these are very explicit scripting processes, as in fitness appraisal, wherein people write detailed workout and dietary plans for themselves, scheduling when they will work out, and at what intensities, and laying out dietary plans for the timing and consumption of proteins, carbohydrates, supplements, and other elements. Prescription can also involve the work of coaches and personal trainers. Computer programs for exercise also participate in this prescriptive process. Less formally and perhaps more insidiously, people may write the future of their desire in the emotional economy that draws on the description and inscription of lack that charts a life of general dissatisfaction and the futuring will to fill that lack in the overall resolve to 'improve' themselves, monitor themselves, and live wherever possible according to the parergonal and instrumental logic of modern efficiency, productivity, and the technological life.

The negative implications of such prescriptions should be evident following my deconstruction of the body that is described by the technology of physical fitness, below. I turn now first to that description of the body and then to the ways in which cults of inscription and prescription insinuate it into everyday life.

Description

Following Heidegger's critique of modern technology, I have argued that puissance is re-sourced such that its connective energy is harnessed by the engines of production and consumption in capitalism. The body, in short, is a resource for the modern economy. This resourcing production of puissance can be aligned with Foucault's analysis of the productivity of biopower – the highly disciplined, active production of life along restrictive political and economic lines. We can also grasp that re-sourcing of puissance via Deleuze's analysis of the territorializing/deterritorializing/reterritorializing of our BwO. As Deleuze and Guattari postulate, capitalism deterritorializes our BwO from the restrictions of 'inherent' codes and recodifies it in the abstraction of value. Capitalism frees desire of its 'inherent' codification in logics such as good and evil and recodifies it according to various logics of value.

Resource management depends on systems of evaluation that code the potential for the sources to be re-sourced in various economic, intellectual, and other cultural projects that can take place only where beings can be marshalled (enframed, *Gestell*) to appear as available for such projects. A forest, for instance, is not available to the resource management of forestry without the intricate evaluating systems that calculate its potential in complex techniques such as extraction, transportation, and marketing, not to mention the more recent practice of evaluating the environmental and contingent political costs of that resource development. Similarly, the body is available as a resource only where there are hermeneutic systems for evaluating and then producing its potential energy. The descriptive practices of the intertextual ensemble of the technology of physical fitness set the hermeneutic context for understanding, evaluating, and developing the body's resource potential. My task here is to deconstruct that context in order to show how those hermeneutic assumptions organize parergonal limits for how the ensemble represents the body.

The evaluation of the body is crucial to each of the five major spheres of the intertextual ensemble. In the texts of government policy, evaluation takes shape, for instance, in terms of calculations of the cost of the lack of physical fitness to the health care system, to general economic productivity, to rates of morbidity, to longevity, and so on. The academic texts calculate values in accordance with the various sciences' particular orientations: aerobic capacity, biomechanics of force, psychological preparedness for performance, and so on. Popular texts assign values to bodies in terms of factors such as age, ratio of fat to lean, intensity of exercise, quantity of exercise, and caloric intake and expenditure. Physical fitness products assign values to establish the 'fit' between particular bodies and particular machines – size, fitness level, age, and so on. Popular representations of the body, while seldom assigning numerical values, describe value in 'qualitative' terms according to such popular conceptions as attractiveness and moral acceptability, whereby the fit body is understood as a sign of a disciplined and productive life. The intelligibility of such valuing of bodies is the product of discourse.

In 'The Order of Discourse,' Foucault (1981) says that discourse works by 'the action of an imposed scarcity, with a fundamental power of affirmation' (73). Discourse subtracts the range of possibility by affirming particular paths of possibility. This understanding of discourse is similar to Deleuze's treatment of the simulacrum: the partial concretization of potential by codes. The various texts of the technology of physical fitness affirm the potential for power over life, in terms of decreased morbidity and in terms of increased longevity, productivity, wellness, self-esteem, physical and emotional capacity, happiness, attractiveness, youthfulness ... An advertisement for a subscription to *Men's Health*, for instance, reads 'Gain Muscle, Lose Fat, More Sex, Better Sex, Get Abs Like These, Mail This Card to Get a Year of *Men's Health*.' I do not deny that following the prescriptions of the texts may increase these increases, although it is difficult to deliver on promises such as those of *Men's Health*. But this affirmation of power over life depends on a *logos* of the body that reproduces the essentially economic organization of reality (in terms of accumulation, expenditure, and accounting) that underlies the other projects of resource management in the modern technological, capitalist order.[1]

The discourse that is set to work in the texts of the technology of physical fitness affirms the potential for humans to seize power over life, by assuming that such power is lacking and that without it life is diminished. The technology of physical fitness affirms the human capacity to overcome the economics of lack by the proper resource management of its energy. This is the discourse that is woven throughout the ensemble and on which its intelligibility depends. Historically deterritorialized of the tyranny of the Christian coding of the inherent fallen nature of 'man,' who can be saved only by divine intervention, the economics of lack reterritorializes our BwO, offering salvation by the resource management of its energy.

Situating the body as a resource management project in the economics of lack makes it available as a resource for the modern capitalist project that reterritorializes desire for the development of production and consumption. The process of inscription impresses the codes of the technology of physical fitness into the flesh of individuals, calling the body to account for its accumulation of value according to the codes of fitness, within the parameters of the various textual fields – for example, aerobic capacity, fat-to-lean ratios, degrees of flexibility, psychological health, sexual desirability, and marketability. As I show below in the section on prescription, the management of the body's desiring energy addresses its lacks through the disciplinary technology of physical fitness. In this way the technology mobilizes desire as a resource for the economics of production and consumption.

Understanding the body as lacking and as in need of strategies to accumulate resources to protect itself against the dangers of lack is, of course, a strikingly familiar way of thinking about the body. Our entire intertextual ensemble assumes that human beings, both as a species and as individuals, can and should take greater control over the production of reality. Increasingly, modern life is conceived as a problem of managing risks (Beck 1992). Risk management, I suggest, is a project of containing the threats that lack of control pose for the human species, nations, economies, communities, and individuals. The calculations of risk management underpin the scientific consensus that physical activity is the greatest single deterrent for the risk of 'all-cause mortality' (Lakka et al. 1994; Lee, Hsieh, and Paffenbarger 1995; Lee and Paffenbarger 2000; Lee, Paffenbarger, and Hennekens 1997; Morris et al. 1980; 1990; Paffenbarger, Kampert, and Lee 1997; Pate et al. 1995; Sesso, Paffenbarger, and Lee 2000; Slattery, Jacobs, and Nichaman 1989; U.S. Department 1996).

The Canadian Fitness and Lifestyle Research Institute (2002), for example, published a 'Warning to Couch Potatoes': 'Almost two-thirds of Canadians are putting themselves at unnecessary risk of early death, heart disease, adult-onset diabetes, colon cancer and other medical conditions because they are not active enough.' They point out the state's interest in controlling this 'risk': 'In August 1997, the federal–provincial/territorial Ministers responsible for fitness, active living, recreation and sport set as a joint target a 10% reduction in the proportion of inactive Canadians over the five-year period from 1998 to 2003. In 1995, the Ministers had already recognized that "physical inactivity represented a major health risk and that physically inactive Canadians were a priority for government action." In 1997, they approved and endorsed "Physical Inactivity: A Framework for Action," a framework detailing the following health, social and economic aims and specific objectives to guide joint actions to reduce physical inactivity (http://www.cflri.ca/cflri/tips/98/LT98_01.html).' Robert Crawford and Bordo have emphasized the moral imperative for control that underpins the culture of physical fitness (Bordo 1993b; Crawford 1984). I argue that there are also cosmological imperatives in this quest for control.

Each of the textual fields of our ensemble represents knowledges and practices that maximize human control. Health promotion strives to control population health, which Foucault has called the biopolitics of the population (Peterson 1997). Academic exercise science produces experimental knowledge by controlling the physical and psychological processes of individual humans and animals in order to determine how to apply its laboratory control over reality outside the lab so as to increase its control over the destiny of human organisms, be it in sport performance or in health. The popular texts of physical fitness write narratives of control for improving cardiovascular health, longevity, body shape and image, mood, self-esteem, sport performance, economic productivity, personal discipline, and so on. Physical fitness products control the body's movements in order to produce the above results. And more subtly, popular representations of the fit body attempt to control the popular imagination of how the body should look.

There is in this quest for control a parergonality of desire that is now foundational to the modern organization of life, which Heidegger has called *Gestell*. The codes of resource management are now so pervasive in modern thinking, they have been so successful in reterritorializing desire, that it is difficult, even terrifying, to imagine living without the codes that facilitate accumulation in the instrumental reason of resource and risk management. It is commonly thought that if we do not rationally manage our resources, both of the earth and of the body, we risk doom. The parergonal logic of resource management suggests the potential for doom and goes to work at building systems that try to avoid it – even though, as the wanton destruction of the ecosphere suggests, this rationality has not yet reached beyond providing for the short-term material comforts of relatively wealthy human beings of the so-called developed and developing worlds. In order to deconstruct the construction of desire in the technology of physical fitness (the codified resource management of the body), we must consider the doom that the technology attempts to avoid. To this end, we look in this section at human sovereignty; its central pillars of humanism and egoism; its denial of death and ageing; its elevation of the self; its construction of the phallic body; and its concept of salvation through accumulations of physical capital.

Human Sovereignty

As Deleuze and Guattari (1983) point out, the repetition of old forms contributes to the reterritorializing of desire that is necessary for capitalism's successful exploitation of the energy of puissance. 'Capitalism institutes or restores all sorts of residual and artificial, imaginary, or symbolic territories, thereby attempting, as best it can, to recode, to rechannel persons who have been defined in terms of abstract quantities' (34–5). The great code – the ancient discourse that is recirculated in many reterritorializations of desire in the modern world, especially in the technology of physical fitness – is the myth that life is constituted by the play of sovereignty. In the Judaeo-Christian ontotheological tradition, this involved the sovereignty of God and the subordination of everything to his divine will. There are, of course, many references to the sovereignty of God in the Bible. The European Enlightenment philosopher and scientist Sir Isaac Newton expresses this myth, arguing that by simple observation we can see God's dominion in everything:

> The most beautiful system of the sun, planets and comets could only proceed from the counsel and dominion of an intelligent and powerful Being ... He is eternal and infinite, omnipotent and omniscient; that is, his duration reaches from eternity to eternity; his presence from infinity to infinity; he governs all things, and knows all things that are or can be done ... We know him only by his most wise and excellent contrivances

of things, and final causes; we admire him for his perfection, but we reverence and adore him on account of his dominion; for we adore him as his servants; and a god without dominion, providence, and final causes is nothing but Fate and Nature. Blind metaphysical necessity, which is certainly the same always and everywhere, could produce no variety of things. All that diversity of natural things which we find suited to different times and place could arise from nothing but the ideas and will of a Being necessarily existing. (Newton 1934)

While still informed by Christian ontotheology, this quotation expresses one of the central myths of modernity inherited from Christianity – the ultimate nature of reality is the product of domination. For Newton that power of domination is God; domination is both the source of reality and the ground for true knowledge of it.

Mark Taylor argues that, with the death of God in the nineteenth and twentieth centuries, dominion was mythically given over to humanity and to the truth-making of modern science. I pursue below the role of domination in the making of truth in the paradigms (Rouse 1987) of the exercise sciences. But I first consider the ways in which the death of the sovereign God and the ascent of sovereign humanity reterritorialize desire in the parergonal logic of domination with a codependent emotional economy of fear. The quest for bodily sovereignty and the fear of sovereign failure contextualize the technology of physical fitness as a quest for power over the body fuelled by fear of the lack of the same. That context makes the intertextual ensemble intelligible and seductive for its readers. The codification of our limitless BwO in the discursively produced economics of scarcity requires a formidable cultural apparatus, one that compels its subjects to read infinity as finite.

Kenneth Surin (1998) says that finitude characterizes the modern *epistèmè*: 'It could be said that prior to the onset of modernity, *infinity* and *perfection* were the primary forces that shaped human beings. Liberation, in this epoch that extended from antiquity until its demise in the European eighteenth century, was understood as the quest for perfection and the transcending of finitude. In modernity, a relatively brief epoch that reached a point of culmination in the European nineteenth century, *finitude* became the primary norm for envisioning the textures of human life' (181).

I suggest that the primacy of human finitude in the health sciences in general and in the technology of physical fitness in particular suggests that that nineteenth-century legacy is still with us. As I argue, the intelligibility of the ensemble depends on an entire modernist cosmology. This cosmology repeats the old myth of the fallen state of humanity. But rather than seeking salvation in the grace of the sovereign, patriarchal God, it points to sovereign selves that pull themselves up by their own finite bootstraps – one of the strategies of which, as we see below, is exercise and diet. It is a cosmology that makes desire conceptually available to the reterritorializing imperatives of pouvoir: the technological construction of desire in an economy of lack constructs the 'need' for fulfilment by technological means, thus plugging desire into the project of resource management. The processes of description and inscription apply this fundamental description of the body to specific, individualized bodies.

In chapter 2, I pointed out that some writers, especially Calvin Luther Martin (1992), have traced this myth to the dawn of the Neolithic, that evolutionary point where humans take control over the production of reality by the development of agriculture and the domestication of animals. I draw briefly on more recent developments in modernity, which, while obviously the inheritors of the domineering neolithic attitude toward 'nature,' bear more specifically on the simulacrum of the subjects of modern life as evidenced in the intertextual ensemble of physical fitness.

The 'death of God' describes in ontotheological terms the transformation of the cosmology of humanity that followed the advent of modern technology in the eighteenth-century industrial revolution. As Taylor (1984) says, 'Social rebellion reflects and is reflected by intellectual revolution' (22). He charts the patricidal intellectual revolution that deposed the theocentric dominion of the Judaeo-Christian God and imposed the anthropocentric dominion of (European) humanity. That revolution, I suggest, provided the conceptual framework for the modern technological re-sourcing (pouvoir) of the source (puissance) of human being that is at work in the technology of physical fitness. The ontotheological tradition described God, the radically other of humanity, as the source of being and of all authentic becoming. In modern technology, in contrast, humanity becomes the ultimate reference point, and being becomes a resource for its projects, both individually and collectively. Descartes's *Cogito ergo sum* expresses this momentous shift in Western thought, grounding reality in human subjectivity. This same subjectivity is the ground of empirical science, wherein human perception is the source of knowledge and the ground for scientifically informed practice. As Heidegger observes, Man becomes the *hypokeimenon*. But this anthropocentric grounding of reality is not the openness of alterity (Cornell 1992; Taylor 1987), the radical freedom for truly empirical encounters with and production of reality (Nancy 1993). Instead it projects a framework of domination for the experience and production of reality.

As Nietzsche writes, 'With the death of God ... released from any fixed centre, everything is left to wander through seemingly infinite space, erring backward, sideward, forward – in all directions' (Taylor 1984, 20). This death marks the deterritorialization of our BwO, freed of the 'inherent' theocentric codes of Christianity. The deterritorialized BwO, however, is reterritorialized by the grounding subjectivity of humanity. Taylor observes that 'modernism ... involves the effort to overturn the hierarchical structures of domination upon which Western thought and society traditionally have rested. As such, it represents a contest both for and against mastery' (20). Human mastery ends up reproducing a similar violent struggle in the perpetual quest for human sovereignty. 'The reversal of divinity and humanity is the distinctive mark of humanistic atheism. Instead of simply denying the reality of God, the humanistic atheist transfers the attributes of the divine to the human self ... By transferring the predicates of divinity to the human subject, the humanistic atheist inverts, but fails to subvert, the logic of repression. With this inversion the problem of mastery and slavery is relocated rather than resolved. The death of the sovereign God now appears to be the birth of the sovereign self' (25).

Humanism and Egoism

Pivotal to the modern sovereign project are humanism and egoism. Humanism names the doctrine by which the (culturally European) human species claims sovereignty. Egoism names the doctrine by which individuals do the same for themselves – although I am arguing that that is its 'ideological' role; egoism actually subjects people to exploitive, reterritorializing discourses. In other words, what looks like freedom is actually the opposite. Modernity turns on the human subject – in the macrocosm, as a species, and in the microcosm, as individuals. Emphasizing the political role of the organization of population (macrocosm) and individuals (microcosm), Foucault refers to these as the bio-politics of the population and the anatamo-politics of the individual, respectively. This cosmology founds the scientific technology of physical fitness: the human species is the foundation of knowledge and centre of practice, and the self is the site of sovereigntist atheistic humanism.

With the modern turn to the subject, there is no longer an attempt at alterity, at trying to be open to what is beyond human subjectivity. Human subjectivity grounds modern cosmology. This cosmology has philosophical dimensions.

In the wake of Descartes's meditations, modern philosophy becomes a *philosophy of the subject*. As the locus of certainty and truth, subjectivity is the first principle from which everything arises and to which all must be returned. With the movement from Descartes, through the Enlightenment to idealism and romanticism, attributes traditionally predicated on the divine subject are gradually displaced onto the human subject. Through a dialectical reversal, the creator God dies and is resurrected in the creative subject. As God created the world through the Logos, so man creates a 'world' though conscious and unconscious projection [which in Heidegger's nomenclature, I have argued, is also a *logos*]. In different terms, the modern subject defines itself by its *constructive* activity. Like God, this sovereign subject relates only to what it constructs and therefore is unaffected by anything other than itself. What appears to be a relationship to otherness – be that other God, nature, objects, subjects, culture or history – always turns out to be an aspect of mediate self-relation that is necessary for complete self-realization in transparent self-consciousness. (Taylor 1987, xxii)

Taylor also stresses the powerful religious underpinnings of this secular modernism:

[There is a] close tie between modern humanistic atheism and its apparent opposite Reformation theology ... Luther started a religious and social revolution by directing theological attention to the individual believer. Plagued by dread, doubt and despair, Luther constantly sought the certainty afforded by a *personal* relationship with God, mediated by Christ. He believed that faith in the free grace of God could provide the security for which believers long. The conclusion of this quest for salvation is summarised succinctly in the theological doctrine implied by the phrase *pro nobis*. The significance of Christ, Luther argued, lies in the 'fact' that he lived and died *'for us'* ... For many people ... the notion that Christ is always *pro nobis* signalled a significant shift toward the central-

ity of the self. From this point of view, the emphasis on individual salvation suggested that *human* concerns lie at the centre of the divine and
therefore cosmic purpose ... This anthropological preoccupation grew
considerably in the years following the reformation. (21)

Humanism is not only a philosophical doctrine that succeeded Christianity. Heidegger (1977) emphasizes that humanism is part of the will
to power of modern technology. 'Within the "framework" (*Gestell*) of
science and technology, natural and human resources appear to be
nothing more than a "standing reserve" open to the manipulation of
powerful agents. Nietzsche's "overman" is the precursor of modern
scientific-technological man who, in his "will to power" or "struggle
for mastery" sets for himself "the task of taking dominion over the
earth"' (92, 96–7). In the absence of the creator God, 'man exalts himself to the posture of lord of the earth [and of himself]. In this way the
impression comes to prevail that everything man encounters exists
only insofar as it is his *construct*. This illusion, in turn, gives rise to one
final delusion: It seems as though man everywhere and always encounters only himself' (27, emphasis added). Such aggressive humanism cuts us off from the rest of reality, resulting in what Thomas Berry
(1988) has called 'cultural autism' – an inability to communicate mean-
ingfully with anything but ourselves.

Heidegger describes the narcissistic anthropocentrism that underlies modern humanism. That anthropocentrism establishes a narcissistic parergonality that renders as second encounters with radical difference – i.e., with that which is not 'human,' the altering difference that
the alter-human holds. This is the problem with academic exercise
science: it is founded on the perceptual apparatus that makes human
subjectivity *the* as structure for any encounter. Thus humanity sets the
parergonality for the technological approach to the body in physical
fitness. Taylor (1984) highlights the philosophical history of the
anthropocentrism of humanist science: 'The empiricism and experi-
mentalism that were necessary for the emergence of modern science
were, in fact, direct outgrowths of the nominalist emphasis on the
significance of the individual and the nominalist insistence on the
essential role of sense experience in the knowing process. As important as this individualism and empiricism, however, was what seemed
to some thinkers to be a scientific analogue to Luther's doctrine of *pro
nobis*. Early scientific investigation argued that all of nature is potentially "for us." In order to realize this potential, the searching scientist

had to put nature "to the rack and compel her [*sic*] to answer our questions" [Francis Bacon's infamous account of experimental science]. From this point of view, the world is intended to respond to human probing and to serve *man's* purposes' (21).

Certainly this is the approach of academic exercise science that does research on rats, for instance, who are regularly 'sacrificed' so that their bodies can be opened to the dominating gaze of science. As I argued above in chapter 1, this science takes place in laboratories, not in observatories: the labour and deaths of the experimental animals used for research on the effects of exercise on metabolism, for example, are expended purely for humanity. The widely accepted assumption that it is ethically acceptable for animals to be *man*ipulated and killed to produce knowledge for the technological advancement of man, attests to this anthropocentric cosmology.

Science based in such humanistic reductionism establishes a parergonality that renders second an alteritous encounter with the reality of movement. That which does not become present in the anthropocentric experiments and calculations of science is not encountered by the science and does not enter into the technology of physical fitness. There are very few texts in our ensemble that explore the alter-human possibilities of the moving body, which I explored in chapter 2 under 'puissance.'[2] So the texts of the exercise sciences give the reader only an encounter with the grounding of humanity. That grounding is the will-to-power, the reality of human domination. The humanist project is exceedingly ambitious. Zygmunt Bauman observes: 'Ambition was to found a human order on earth, in which freedom and happiness prevailed, without any transcendental or supernatural supports – an entirely human order ... To place man at the centre meant he had to become the Archimedean point around which everything revolved ... The axiom on which the humanist rock was to be forged was put as well by Pico della Mirandola in 1486 as by anyone: "We can become what we will" ... So the humanist fathers put their founding axiom: man is all-powerful, if his will is strong enough. He can create himself. He can choose to be courageous, honourable, just, rich, influential, or not' (Carroll 1993, 2–3, as cited in Bauman 1998, 61).

Bauman adds: 'Contrary to Carroll's suggestion that the humanist creed drew inspiration from Archimedes, who believed that he stole the secrets of the gods, it rather turned Protagoras's contemplative idea that "man is the measure of all things" into a declaration of practical intent' (61). The idea that humanity can create itself, perhaps not endlessly, but at least to some degree, is a theme that appears in all the texts of our ensemble; the very idea of physical training assumes such power of self-creation. The practical intention of the technology is to create more powerful, in the sense of pouvoir, human subjects.

Frequently lauded as an improvement over the structures of domination that were part of Judaeo-Christian theism, humanism actually reproduces such structures. It operates like the other -isms that are now widely criticized – racism, sexism, classism, ablism, ageism, and so on. Some have criticized humanism for its pretence to a concept of a universal humanity, which is in fact the projection of white, European, modern, male humanity onto the rest of the world. From an ecospherical perspective, which in chapter 2 I argued is the perspective of puissance, it is also anthropocentric. John Hodge (1990) suggests that underlying these -isms is the problem of duality based on hierarchies: 'In Western societies dualist justifications typically take a particular form as a consequence of the identification of good with reason, law and rationality, and bad with emotion, chance, spontaneity, and nature. In accordance with this form of dualism, control of nature through science and technology is generally assumed to be good. This assumption determines the very meaning Western nations attach to the concept of "civilization." The development of societies from "primitive" to "civilized" is often equated with the development of the tools and technological devices that can be used to control nature. Development means technological, industrial and scientific progress' (96–7).

The dualism of humanism insinuates a parergonal logic of human mastery. It involves, of course, the technological mastery of non-human nature: other animals, plants, rivers, and so on. This centrality of humans has a long history in Western culture: 'The social and moral traditions that have been dominant in the West ... have not involved the idea that animals, trees, or the land in their own right, as distinct from their owners or their Creator, have moral standing. Only a few saints and reformers have taught that people have direct moral responsibility to nonhuman creatures' (Rockefeller 1992). Modern humanism is the crystallization of this historical anthropocentrism. 'The humanist pushes to its conclusive Cartesian *reductio ad hominem* by attempting to humanize the entire world. Freed from the Creator God, the creative subject engages in "calculative thinking," which views "the world as our own, our private property, designed according to our needs and readily domesticated" (Robbe-Grillet 1965, p. 24)' (Taylor 1984, 26). Humanist mastery also involves dominion over the 'nature' of human beings. Calculative mastery over the uncontrolled nature of the body is the project of the technology of physical fitness – as I showed above, calculation is characteristic of the technology in all the fields, some more arithmetically than others. That 'nature' is nothing 'natural'; it is the lack that must always appear wherever there is the socially constructed desire for sovereignty.

We are not, of course, sovereign. Change, death, and decay are always ultimately sovereign. Fear of that ultimate doom is what the texts of the technology of physical fitness promise to control, if the human subject will submit to the resource management of the technology. Humanistic dualism fashions the essential impermanence of movement (the essence of being/becoming) as the negative other that needs to be controlled. While the technology of physical fitness does not maintain the fantasy that change, death, and decay can ultimately be overcome – high-technology genetic modification science and computer science play with *that* sovereigntist hope – it does construct their advent as a failure of sovereignty that can be postponed. Sovereign success, at least at this point of technological development, is necessarily partial. This parergonality therefore attempts to bring some stasis to life and to render impermanence second. As such, it reproduces the Christian desire for stasis expressed in a famous nineteenth-century English hymn that is popular at funerals: 'Abide with me; fast falls this eventide; / The darkness deepens, Lord with me abide ... / Change and decay in all around I see; / O thou who changest not, abide with me' (Monk 1933).

Uncertainty and fear of it permeate the modern egocentric subject. Taylor (1984) explores the philosophical expression of this: 'Descartes, like his theological precursor, Luther suffered nearly pathological doubt. Descartes's entire philosophical enterprise can be understood as an effort to overcome the insecurity brought about by uncertainty and to reach the security promised by certainty. Suspecting that the hand that inflicts the wound holds the cure, Descartes radicalized doubt. He doubted everything until he discovered that which is unconditionally indubitable – the *cogito*. Then, in a move destined to change the earth, Descartes identified truth with certainty. Truth, in other words, is *pro nobis* ... The identification of truth with certainty is, in effect, a *reductio ad hominem*. When fully developed, the Cartesian philosophy of the *cogito* leads to the "theory of the subject," which lies at the heart of humanism' (22).

The *pro nobis* (for us) that is the atheistic humanist inheritance of Luther's soteriology is also *pro me* (for me). As an anthropocentric enterprise, humanism posits the dominion of humanity at the centre of its cosmology. Egocentrism brings, as Foucault would say, 'greater resolution' to that cosmology by making the individual human subject and sense of self the centre of concern, the number-one project. All the textual fields of physical fitness centre on the individual. As I showed above in chapter 3, even the texts on population health focus on the individual, which, as Foucaultian critiques of health care have maintained, is the pre-eminent site of disciplinary control for the population as a whole (Peterson and Bunton 1997). In the descriptive workings of the intertextual ensemble, egocentrism marks the hermeneutic context; in the work of inscription and prescription, it marks the site of practice.

The ego is a fragile territorialization of puissance – forever at risk of losing its ground, giving way to the discombobulation of change, decay, and death, it is 'at risk' of following the movement of life itself. The death of the sovereign God, the ensuing, inverted quest for human sovereignty, and uncertainty in the face of that search led to the project of modern subject formation, which is the struggle, for stasis, control. The sovereign quest territorializes the smooth space of movement, producing striated spaces through which movement is managed as a resource for the modern subject. The infinite difference that smooth space potentializes is territorialized by the modern subject, which needs to control space in order to gain sovereignty. The altering difference that change, decay, and death offer the modern subject is that which it most firmly rejects. Invoking Hegel's analysis of the master–slave relationship, Taylor describes the subjectivity that is born in the death of God: 'In an effort to overcome alienation and gain self-possession, slave rebels against master and son turns against father. The subversive activity of the subject has as its goal mastery of the master. By overthrowing the lord, the subject hopes to establish identity, maintain integrity, and protect propriety (as well as property). This struggle for mastery joins affirmation and negation. The self asserts itself by negating the other, which it regards in thoroughly negative terms. Consequently, the rebellious subject embodies a form of negation in which identity secures itself by *excluding* difference. Instead of subverting the "logic" of mastery, this negative activity merely turns it to its own ends... The servile subject tries to master the terror that absolute alterity provokes by negating the wholly other and enclosing the self within the secure "solitude of solidarity and self-identity"' (Taylor 1984, 24, with quote from Derrida (1978, 91)).

Rejecting Death and Ageing

The negation of otherness in the production of identity is the parergonal logic for the territorializing of the modern subject. Death is the ultimate depravity, the 'wholly other,' the terrifying, absolute difference to identity that constitutes the modern subject. 'Identity secures itself by *excluding* difference' (Taylor 1984, 24). The modern fear of death is the fear of the cosmology of sovereign subjectivity being undermined. As such it is the fear of the loss of the ultimate nature of Western reality, which, as Newton articulated, is domination. 'Faced with the absolute fear brought about by the encounter with the wholly other, "man precisely as the one so threatened, exalts himself to the posture of lord of the earth. In this way the impression comes to prevail that everything man encounters exists only insofar as it his construct"' (Taylor 1984, 25, with quote from Heidegger 1977, 27).

Where the body itself becomes the construct of the human subject, as it does in the technology of physical fitness, its decay and demise are testimony to the inevitable ultimate failure of sovereign individuality.[3] The human subject, created by the larger modern technological project as the ongoing design of individual self-creation in the quest to establish security in identity, fearfully excludes the difference that change, decay, and death promise. In this way, the essentially impermanent movement of the body becomes the negative other that needs to be erased by the more stable identity of the physically fit: the technologically physically fit body is one that dominates the movement of life. This means that the popular image of the lean, youthful, and buff body signifies sovereignty. It is an essentially negative image; grasping for stasis, it says 'NO' to the difference that the movement of life presents. Alterity, with its openness to difference, and change, which includes embracing death and yielding to our profound lack of control, are absolutely at odds with the modern logic of domination.

We can see the intolerability of death to the modern subject in the relative disappearance of death as a public phenomenon. Zygmunt Bauman (1988) writes: 'Death has become a somewhat shameful and embarrassing affair, somewhat akin to pornography (as Geoffrey Gorer [1965] observed), an event not to be discussed in public and certainly "not in front of the children." The dead and particularly the dying have been removed beyond the confines of daily life, assigned separate spaces not accessible to the public, and entrusted to the care of "professionals." The elaborate and spectacular public ceremony of funerals has been replaced with the brief and on the whole private event of the burial or incineration of the body under the efficient supervision of the experts' (65).

We can note the disappearance of death also in the increasingly popular minimalist public rituals, where they are even held, called 'Celebrations of Life,' rather than requiems or funerals.

This embarrassment about death, I suggest, is the embarrassment of failed sovereignty. Taylor (1987) writes of Derrida's deconstruction of the modernist grand systems for erasing death, silencing its knell. To reproduce its fantasy, the modernist sovereign quest requires such silence about death. The technology of physical fitness is part of the project (along with a host of other strategies): marshalling the forces of life, it tries to muffle the clap of death, the shattering significance, the terrible tear, that death inevitably makes in the push for the sovereignty of the human ego. The disappearance of death affirms the *appearance* of human sovereignty.

I wrote above that the inevitability of death makes success with the technology of physical fitness necessarily partial. Death occurs, but it disappears in the modern minimalist 'rituals' that surround it. Death also disappears in the technological approach to avoiding it. According to Bauman (1998): '[Death] is now dissolved in the minute, yet innumerable traps and ambushes of daily life. One tends to hear it knocking now and again, in fatty fast foods, in listeria-infected eggs, in cholesterol-rich temptations, in sex without condoms, in cigarette smoke, in asthma-inducing carpet mites, in the "dirt you see and germs you do not," in over-eating and over-dieting, in too much ozone content and the hole in the ozone layer; but one knows how to barricade the door when death knocks, and one can always replace the old and rusty locks and bolts and alarms with "new and improved ones"' (65).

The technology of physical fitness mans the barricades of death, always working its market for 'new and improved' technological innovations. (The discourse of the 'new and improved' is one of the primary engines of scientific research in health.) Dealing with death becomes a technical matter of dealing 'innovatively' with these little knocks at the door. Bauman's point is that this focus on managing particular risks trivializes the enormity of death.

The philosophy of the limit takes Bauman's observation further. By systematically controlling for various possible deaths, the technology claims increasing sovereignty for humans over their destiny. For the canny technologist, death becomes pre-eminently a management problem. Such management can erase particular deaths' otherness. The technology of physical fitness, for instance, describes the body as being at risk of various deadly threats that can and should be managed strategically through the calculated use of exercise and diet. Erasing the ultimate risk of death is beyond its power. But where death is divided up, as it were, into various risk factors, death becomes a manageable problem. With the right strategy, for instance, one can avoid dying of atherosclerosis. This establishes sovereignty over a particular cause of death. A highly successful management strategy will avoid a whole range of deathly scenarios. Death's range thus appears limited, more and more under the control of technological humans. For the technology of physical fitness, the focus of life is avoidance of death. Its message is to live by attempting to erase death.

In such a life, death should start to disappear. But it doesn't. It is for ever present as the silenced, threatening other, the very terror of which forces one into a technologically managed life. This is decidedly not an alteritous attitude towards death. Under technology, death itself becomes striated, a negatively energized resource for channelling people into the modern technological way of being. The threat of death becomes a strategy of pouvoir. In this way, the seeming disappearance of death is actually the invisible negative energy that produces a particular way (striation) of life. The sovereignty of this technological life, ironically enough, turns out to be the sovereignty of death. The seeming disappearance of death in modernity actually marks its power (pouvoir). The secondness of death in the parergonality of the modern technology of physical fitness is essential to the system!

In the alterity of compassionate emptiness, in contrast, death is not a threat but a powerful promise of difference, a genuine openness to which allows for a fearless life, lived in the smooth space of which death is a part. In the practice of emptiness, death is neither sought nor aggressively avoided. Thus, in alterity, neither death nor the human subject has dominion. In technology, however, death is the invisible, fearful, panoptic hand that keeps people plugged into the system.

The modern cult of fear has Christian roots. Jean Delumeau (1990) has argued that fear was a major engine of the late medieval and early modern Christian religious culture that spread from the monasteries into the wider populace through forms of preaching and iconography that dwelled on the macabre as an enticement into Christian piety and into the quest for salvation from a horrible after-life of eternal damnation. Delumeau called this 'the evangelism of fear.' 'The insistence on the macabre, in the wake of the *contemptus mundi*, thus stood within a logic of a vast enterprise of guilt-infliction aimed toward salvation and the afterlife' (112–13). The technology of physical fitness appeals to a modern macabre – the damnation that the lack of sovereignty, the guilty decay of the body, the abjection of death, and the ignominy of being physically unfit, of being a poor resource, pose for the modern subject. This modern evangelism of fear is promulgated in government campaigns of health promotion, fitness appraisal, the scientific texts on the risk of not exercising and monitoring diet, exercise journals and exercise regimens, and advertisements that idealize youth and slenderness. In all these, the macabre spectre of human failing, insufficiency, and lack arouses the guilt that makes it all too clear that one must seek salvation from the abyss through the technology of physical fitness.

Now, one might assume that fear and avoidance of death are universal human phenomena. But there are many examples of alteritous comportment towards death. Walt Whitman, for example, sang about the goodness of death in his 1865 poem 'When Lilacs Last in the Dooryard Bloom'd' (verse 14): 'Come lovely and soothing death, / Undulate round the world, serenely arriving, arriving, / In the day, in the night, to all, to each, / Sooner or later delicate death. / Prais'd be the fathomless universe, / For life and joy, and for objects and knowledge curious, / And for love, sweet love – but praise! praise! praise! / For the sure-enwinding arms of cool-enfolding death.'

And Rilke speaks similarly of death as an intimate companion, a 'friend': 'We should not be afraid that our strength is insufficient to endure any experience of death, even the closest and most terrifying. Death is not *beyond* our strength; it is the measuring-line at the vessel's brim: we are *full* whenever we reach it – and being full (for us) means being heavy. – I am not saying that we should *love* death; but we should love life so generously, so without calculation and selection, that we involuntarily come to include, and to love death too (life's averted half); this is in fact what always happens in the great turmoils of love, which cannot be held back or defined. Only because we exclude death, when it suddenly enters our thoughts, has it become more and more of a stranger to us; and because we have kept it a stranger, it has become our enemy. It is conceivable that it is infinitely closer to us than life itself' (1989, 331). Prejudice, Rilke writes, distorts our image of death: 'It is a *friend*, our deepest friend, perhaps the only one who can never be misled by our attitudes and vacillations – and this, you must understand, *not* in the sentimental-romantic sense of life's opposite, a denial of life: but here, to living and working on earth, to Nature, to love. Life simultaneously says Yes and No. Death (I implore you to believe this) is the true Yes-sayer. It says *only* Yes. In the presence of eternity' (332).

Both Whitman and Rilke express the potential for alterity – a profound openness to otherness that allows it to change us. Death is an enemy when we are so afraid of life that we fear its thresholds, fear the altering power of going beyond boundaries, fear, in short, puissance. Pouvoir keeps the otherness of death at a distance. For pouvoir, death is the panoptic line that should not be crossed. It is the unimaginable other that keeps the living living within the structures of modern panoptic selfhood, the centre of which is sovereignty, identity, self-preservation in the face of otherness. As Taylor wrote above, 'The self asserts itself by negating the other, which it regards in thoroughly negative terms.' The modern technological project of resource management represents the enervation of death: it has no value, use, or meaning. The modern technological self therefore asserts itself by regarding death in thoroughly negative terms. From the perspective of modernity, death marks not the fulfilment of life, which Rilke (1996) metaphorically calls a distillation. 'And here we have Death; a bluish distillate / in a cup without a saucer.'

For modern, egocentric humanity, death is the ultimate de-centring, the dissolution of the modern cosmology that killed God and fatally erected humanity in his place. Death has become failure, failure of human sovereignty. The culture of physical fitness, for instance, exhorts people to exercise to avoid dying of 'heart failure' – a failure that realizes the body's lack of sovereignty. That the heart's stopping is termed a failure is significant. Alternatively, it could be called perhaps life's 'climax,' 'completion,' 'conclusion,' 'turning point,' or the 'brim of the cup of life.' The word 'failure' marks the body in the *functional* project of resource management. More ambitious than the technology of physical fitness, the technology of genetics entertains the fantasy that genetic manipulation will ultimately overcome death. In this egocentric fantasy, the domination of humanity will be complete. Death will be completely negated, the otherness of life thoroughly erased.

Modern death is doubly dark: it connotes not only failure to achieve sovereignty with the energy of *pouvoir*; it also marks the failure to live fearlessly in the alterity of *puissance*. Rilke (1996) adds: 'What sort of beings are these, then, / who finally must be frightened off with poison? ... This hard present moment has to be pulled out / of them like a set of false teeth' (113).

And from non-Western experience, Calvin Luther Martin (1992), for instance, suggests that fear was not the experience of death for North American Indians before the European invasions. He says that their cosmology was profoundly open to ontological change: this is reflected in the many myths of metamorphosis, where various animals and humans changed from one to another. Death was part of the ongoing metamorphosis of life. Metamorphosis means changing forms. A metamorphic cosmology accepts the changing forms of life, embraces difference, including ageing and death, as the essential way of life. It is a non-violent acceptance of impermanence.

Buddhism also embraces impermanence as the nature of life and death. Fulfilment comes not from attachment to life, but from letting go of body and mind. Grasping at life in the face of death, from a Buddhist perspective, causes suffering. Relief comes from egoless transcendence, going beyond life and death. This is traditionally called *prajana paramita*, which is the wisdom (*prajna*) of 'having arrived at the other shore' (*paramita*). Hui-Neng (1998) explains: 'If you understand the meaning, you detach from birth and death. If you fixate on objects, birth and death occur, as when water has waves – this is called "this shore." When you detach from objects, there is no birth or death as when water flows smoothly – this is called "the other shore," so it is referred to as *paramita*, (18). At the other shore, 'Everything is one, the one is everything. Going and coming freely, the substance of mind without blockage' (17). In this wisdom, the coming and going of life and death are neither fearful nor ultimately real.

Annie Dillard (1982) writes: 'I would like to learn, or remember, how to live ... : open to time and death painlessly, noticing everything, remembering nothing, choosing the given with a fierce and pointed will' (68–9).

Modern death's failing and risky companion is ageing. While ageing does not present the complete difference to the modern ego that death does, it is nevertheless a threat to sovereignty. The intertextual ensemble of physical fitness conceptualizes the ageing post-adolescent body as deteriorating; it 'loses' the strength, the flexibility, and the erection that make its bodily sovereignty possible. For the techno-culture of physical fitness, ageing is the decay of youthfulness. The 'natural process of ageing' produces lacks: diminished aerobic capac-ity, less mobility, reduced vitality, less desirability, declining strength. Standard textbooks show graphs of the ageing process in terms of those various functions. There is an increase in the early years after birth and decline in the later.

The technology of physical fitness promises to flatten the descend-ing line in the graph, retarding the decline. This representation has parallels with the accounting graphs that corporations use to chart the growth and decline of financial capital. After a period of prosperous accumulation of physical fitness capital (often quite a short period), the capital is depleted and the individual, like a badly managed cor-poration, begins to fail. The *Oxford English Dictionary* defines decay as 'the process of falling off from a prosperous or thriving condition; progressive decline; the condition of one who has thus fallen off or declined.' The ageing, decaying body marks the individual's fall from sovereignty. Extended youthfulness is one of the promised products of the technology of physical fitness; it promises to perpetuate sover-eignty in the face of its growing lack. The popular texts, products, and representations of physical fitness are blatant in this regard, promis-ing a 'more youthful you.' While government policies and academic texts are more subtle about perpetuating youthfulness and acknowl-edge the inevitability of the 'decline' that comes with ageing for those who continue to live, they do nevertheless posit increased youthful-ness for the ageing as a valuable product of the technology of physical fitness, referring often to 'retarding the effects of old age by exercise and controlled diet,' for example. Ageing, which is essential to living, is a risk to living, ironically enough. Ageing then is constituted discur-sively as a *lack* of youthfulness. Part of the sovereign quest therefore involves the reproduction and accumulation of youthfulness. One may get older, but one should feel, look, act, and function young.

The fear of the difference that ageing presents reflects the desire for stasis that I mentioned above with reference to the hymn 'Abide with me.' It is a fear of the alterity that is presented in the impermanence of the movement of life itself. Recalling Nancy's call for radical world-shattering encounters with ungrounded experience, I suggest that grasping at youth is an attempt to secure a ground in the face of the ultimate lack of ground that the impermanence of aging realizes. Youth-centrism is in short a fear of the freedom that a radical *experience* of ageing, indeed of life, affords.

The Centred Self

The cosmology of the technology of physical fitness is human-, ego-, and youth-centred. It attempts to maintain these centres by dominating that which is off-centre: non-human, non-ego, aged. It does so by objectifying the body.

The academic exercise sciences explicitly objectify the body; in experimental settings they dominate it by controlled movements and measurements that force it to emit signs of its objectification – VO_2max., speed, force, range of flexibility, and so on. Exercise psychology also sees the body primarily as an object that can facilitate or obstruct the dynamics of the self in terms of 'self-concept,' 'self-esteem,' and 'self-efficacy,' for instance. Similarly, the popular texts of physical fitness objectify the body in order to make it more productive for the self, in terms of body shaping, strength, and fitness, as well as motivational strategies to get resistant bodies to exercise more. The products of physical fitness, such as fitness appraisals and exercise equipment such as heart rate monitors, offer objective calculations of individual bodies' productivity to the projects of self-creation and self-preservation. The self becomes the subject, and the body becomes the object that needs to be controlled through the technology of physical fitness in the service of that subject.

Like Taylor, Drucilla Cornell (1992) believes that this is destructive: 'The subject–object relationship necessarily gives rise to the master–slave dialectic. The master–slave dialectic is played out in our relations with nature, taken here to mean both against the external world of things, and against our internal "nature" as physical, sexual beings. Ultimately, the master–slave dialectic takes its toll. The thinking subject's striving for mastery turns against itself. The part of our humanness that is "natural" – sexual desire, our longing for warmth and comfort – succumbs to a rationality whose mission is to drive into submission an essential part of what we are. The subject itself becomes objectified, an object among other objects' (14). This 'essential part of who we are,' I suggest, while it includes 'sexual desire, our longing for warmth and comfort,' is also the fact of the radical impermanence of the body, expressed in its essential movement. The exercise sciences, by objectifying the body, plug it into the master–slave relationship that makes the body's own essence (the impermanence of its moving) radically other to itself, something to be avoided. They objectify the free (smooth) space of our BwO in order to secure a more powerful identity for the master-self who masters the smooth space of movement in order to project itself. This is pouvoir appropriating puissance. The objectifications of the intertextual ensemble form the conceptual framework that makes the domination of puissance possible and available as a resource for pouvoir.

The cosmological *inversion* rather than *subversion* of the slavish, historical relationship between God and humans reproduces in the body a profound negativity of subject and object. Nietzsche (1956), in the *Genealogy of Morals,* writes that the 'slave revolt' is not 'a triumphant affirmation' but a reaction that 'begins by saying *no* to an "outside," an "other," a non-self, and this *No* is its creative act' (171). The death of a sovereign God, replaced by the inverted birth of the sovereign self, perpetuates the logics of domination, in which the dominating parergonality of denial continues to subject the puissance of desire. In Deleuza's terms, it is the reterritorialization of our BwO by the imposition of the sovereign self, which insists on domination for its existence. From the perspective of the philosophy of the limit, the *no* of sovereignty establishes the cosmological parergonality that renders second the openness, the smooth space of movement. It denies the decentring, deterritorializing openness of movement in favour of the closure that secures the pouvoir of anthropocentrism, egocentrism, and youthcentrism, which striates the smooth space of movement (puissance). The alteritous smooth space of movement, in contrast, realizes the Body of Reality, which Dōgen calls 'One Bright Pearl.' In chapter 2, I spoke of Glass's analogy between the myth of Indra's Net and particle and wave theories of light:

Perhaps Indra's Net is better visualized not only as a net of interconnected particle-selves but also as a wave of brilliant light. This wave of light is not static but moves, and exerts a 'force' upon the particle-selves. The net as a whole then takes on the characteristics of the force of the larger wave. Wave, then, embraces particle, but particle does not embrace wave. Seeing the net as light does not negate its particle nature, nor does seeing the light as a set of interconnected particles negate its wave nature – once the action of the wave upon particle is realized. Following this analogue through to the end, the goal of practice [of enlightened desire] would then be to dwell upon one's 'particle-nature' while realizing 'wave-nature' is primary and governs behaviour. This requires not only a shift in focus from particle to wave but a shift in the mode of awareness that guides action, from particle sensitivities to wave sensitivities. (Glass 1995, 78)

The centrisms of the modern humanist cosmology, which ground the technology of physical fitness, render second the wave sensitivities. The modern perspective of the centred subject allows only the particle sensitivities to play. The texts' focus on the individual, and the scientific epistemology that grounds knowledge in human subjectivity, call on only our particulate capacity and omit the profoundly interconnected wave potential from their world picture (Heidegger 1938). Our profound interdependence disappears in this description of us.

The negative logic of domination continues in the mastery of the self that physical fitness expresses as a mode of self creation/perpetuation, which it exploits in the fear of the loss of self, the loss of control that ageing and death threaten. The texts of the technology use death and decay rhetorically, via a device called cataplexis, which tries to convince the reader to accept the texts' cosmological description of the body by threatening misfortune if the reader does not heed the ensemble's message. For example, a professor at the University of Missouri–Columbia has invented a pathology, 'sedentary death syndrome,' to describe those who are not exercising enough.

Fear of sovereign failure is the emotional weave of the modern humanist cosmology. The texts of the technology of physical fitness would make no emotional sense, they would have very little appeal, if they could not exploit this modernist fear of difference. The energy of risk management is the power of fear. The widespread promotion of exercise and fitness reasserts the cultural logic of fear and domination in the face of the profound failure of modernity to deliver on its promise of control. Emptiness faces the alterity of absence fearlessly; it compassionately loves the body's impermanence. Human sovereignty, in contrast, finds its energy precisely by imagining that which is not self as abject:

The abject has only one quality of the object – that of being opposed to I ... If the object, however, through its opposition, settles me within the fragile texture of a desire for meaning, which, as a matter of fact, makes me ceaselessly and infinitely homologous to it, what is *abject*, on the contrary, the jettisoned object, is radically excluded and draws me toward the place where meaning collapses. A certain 'ego' that merged with its master, a superego, has flatly driven it away. It lies outside, beyond the set, and does not seem to agree with the latter's rules of the game ... A massive and sudden emergence of uncanniness, which, familiar as it might have been in an opaque and forgotten life, now harries me as radically separate, loathsome. Not me. Not that. But not nothing either. A "something" that I do not recognize as a thing. A weight of meaninglessness, about which there is nothing insignificant, and which crushes me. On the edge of non-existence and hallucination, of a reality that, if I acknowledge it, it annihilates me. There, abject and abjection are my safeguards. The primers of my culture. (Kristeva 1982, 1–2)

The non-self that death and decay threaten is the 'meaninglessness,' the abjection, that the failure of sovereignty presents to the striated desire of the centred self. The loathsomeness of the non-existence of self is the fear that fuels the technological project of physical fitness. Fear permeates the intertextual ensemble; fear-mongering is its primary commerce. It expresses the fear of lack of control in a variety of ways. For government policy documents, there is the fear of high palliative medical costs that the technologically unfit will draw on the public accounts. Governments also fear the decreased productivity of an unfit workforce – inadequate human resources for the engines of capital production. Fear powers the academic sports sciences as well: here it is the desire to win in competitive sport and the concomitant fear of losing that motivate scientists and funding bodies to develop physical training technologies that decrease the risk of failure in competitive sport. For the health-oriented exercise physiological sciences, fears of mortality and morbidity inspire research. Exercise psychology calls on fear of psychological abnormality or deviance, as well as fear of the looming lacks that the discipline of psychology produces – lack of self-esteem, self-efficacy, self-mastery, self-concept, and so on. The popular texts of physical fitness explicitly capitalize on the fear of lack of control – poor health, ageing, and mortality. And certainly the fear of 'ugliness' is one of the major fuels for physical fitness, where people spend many hours each week exercising in order to maintain or improve their marketability in a culture that values accumulation of physical cultural capital in the accounting systems in such forms as leanness and muscularity.

Abject fear occurs in the face of difference – the not-self. Kristeva (1982) speaks of the abjection of death. While she does not use the term 'sovereignty,' she does speak of death as a 'fall': 'The corpse (or cadaver: *cadere*, to fall), that which has irremediably become a cropper, is cesspool, and death; it upsets even more violently the one who confronts it as fragile and fallacious. A wound with blood and pus, or the sickly, acrid smell of sweat, of decay, does not *signify* death. In the presence of signified death – a flat encephalograph, for instance – I would understand, react or accept. No, as in true theatre, without makeup or masks, refuse and corpses *show me* what I permanently thrust aside in order to live ... There, I am at the border of my condition as a living being. My body extricates itself, as being alive, from that border ... [In death] I behold the breaking down of a world that has erased its borders, fainting away (3–4).

The self is constituted by its territorial borders, by the organization of our BwO. Abjection arises in the fear of the loss of borders. 'It is thus not lack of cleanliness or health that causes abjection but what disturbs identity, system, order' (Kristeva 1982, 4). The technology of physical fitness promises to keep intact the identity, system, and order of the modern self. It pretends to protect the borders of the humanist sovereignty. The self itself can become abject when it realizes that its very identity is produced by the ways in which its borders have cut it off from the infinity of being, which I discussed above in the myth of Indra's Net, the One Bright Pearl, the infinitely interdependent reflecting body, the Body of Reality. 'The abjection of self would be the culminating form of that experience of the subject to which it is revealed that all its objects are based merely on the inaugural *loss* that laid the foundations of its own being' (Kristeva 1982, 5). Humanist sovereignty is therefore the product of loss of connection. Loss and fear thus constitute modern subjectivity. The texts of the ensemble are meaningful because they summon the abjection of modern subjectivity by assuming the necessity of avoiding the horror of the loss of self entailed in the collapse of sovereignty.

The Phallic Body

I have been deconstructing the cosmology of the technology of physical fitness for its anthropocentrism. I now argue that there is a gendered dimension to that anthropocentrism. Like most modern technologies, physical fitness has been overwhelmingly the product of men. Many feminist critiques of science and technology have spoken of the marginality of women in the work of science and technology. Just as atheistic humanism has inherited the logic of domination that operated in the sovereignty of God, so too science and technology have inherited the sexism of Christian clerical culture. Academic science emerged out of the exclusively male Christian monasteries that eventually became the modern universities (Noble 1992). Modern technology is a historically masculine enterprise; women have until very recently been almost entirely excluded from work in science and technology.

While more women are now involved in this culture, the modes of technological manipulation and knowledge production with which both sexes work remain relatively unchanged by the increased participation of women. As I mentioned above, there are a few feminist challenges in the academic sciences of physical fitness, most notably in history and sociology and to a much lesser degree in psychology. The 'hard' sciences – physiology and biomechanics, for instance – have been generally immune to feminist critiques of science. Women's health and fitness are increasingly coming to address important issues, but only within the masculinist paradigms of scientific knowledge, which I maintain are the scientific manifestation of the domineering phallocentrism of modern technology's cosmology of the body. The technology of physical fitness is phallocentric not only because men have dominated it, but also because it expresses the quintessential formation of the modern desire for sovereignty: phallic desire, whose emotional energy is loss and fear.

Phallic desire moves in the opposite direction to emptiness. It is a formation of desire that secures the anthropocentric and egocentric self, conquering difference in the constant struggle for dominating self-preservation. The erect penis is traditionally considered the quintessential embodiment of the phallic will. The more space it commands, the more powerfully phallic it is considered. But the erect penis is but one embodiment of phallic energy. While it is a form of desire that is encouraged among those who have penises and discouraged by those who 'lack' them, the phallus, as an aggressive will to power, is not confined to persons with penises, as Mark Taylor points out. I have argued elsewhere that it is a form of desire that takes considerable training. Competitive sport, traditionally the preserve of men, is part of the education of the phallic will (Pronger 1998; 1999). The success of contemporary women in competitive sport proves that you do not need a penis to exercise phallic desire. And the reluctance of the male-controlled sports media complex to acknowledge that success points to the resentment that people with penises harbour for those who are successfully phallic without them.

The cultures of sport and physical fitness have traditionally discouraged women from being as phallic as men. They have encouraged women to have smaller bodies, to be less aggressive in sport, weaker, more passive. This is still largely the case, as we can see in the epidemic of anorexia among women (Bordo 1993b; Hesse-Biber 1996; Lelwica 1999; Markula 1995; Seid 1989), the many discouragements to girls' participation in physical activity, the marginal media coverage of women's sports, and continued violence against women in general. Women are usually represented as weaker versions of the sovereign male, even though on average they live longer.

The more 'progressive' elements of the culture of physical fitness and sport encourage women to be equally as phallic as men: to play sport the same way, to build muscles the same way, to occupy space the same way. Within the ensemble there is considerable variation in this regard. While the ensemble describes a variety of differences between men and women, in terms of the centrisms of humanism and youthism, it nevertheless presents women as belonging to the same modern sovereign project as men. Self-centrism is represented as more complex for women: their traditional role as caregivers continues to be a feature, and popular texts of the ensemble distinctly organize much of female desirability in terms of the heterosexual male gaze and the 'need' for women to shape their bodies in order to snare a male partner.

And the traditional preoccupation with women's reproductive function also continues to inform much of the science of physical fitness – most exercise physiology textbooks, for instance, have a chapter on the reproductive physiology of females, but not of males. That focus on female reproductive physiology represents a traditional patriarchal cultural understanding of women's bodies being about more than themselves – this is, of course, the argument made by anti-abortion crusaders. The more 'liberated' of the texts in the ensemble, however, represent women as just as self-centred as men.

The technology of physical fitness conceives the entirety of every body as a phallic project. The body should be as erect, firm, independent, and impermeable as possible. While the intertextual ensemble represents both men and women's bodies as phallic in this way, there are important differences between them. Liz Grosz's work on the supposed 'leakiness' of women's bodies, for instance, indicates the challenge that women present to the phallic project of patriarchal control (Grosz and Probyn 1995, 108ff). The idea reproduces the traditional patriarchal understanding of women's bodies being more out of control than men's. Susan Bordo writes about the prevalence of the notion that women need to get control of themselves. She also says that the corollary is that whereas women are supposed to get control over themselves, men are supposed to get control over others. I largely agree with this concept, but I would say that the logic of the phallic domination of the self affects both sexes. It expects men to expand their control to others, but women to limit control to themselves. And there is also considerable variation in the ways in which different texts and fields represent men and women's bodies in the intersections of other discursive matrices, such as race, class, and age. The phallic body can take many shapes in accordance with different discourses: buff, skinny, anorexic, megorexic, feminine, masculine, and so on. But there is a phallocentrism underlying all these variations in the ensemble.

As numbers of feminist writers have argued, phallocentrism amounts to the erasure of women. According to Judith Butler (1990): 'Irigaray clearly suggests that both marker and marked are maintained within a masculinist mode of signification in which the female body is "marked off," as it were, from the domain of the signifiable. In post-Hegelian terms she is "cancelled" but not preserved. On Irigaray's reading, Beauvoir's claim that woman "is sex" is reversed to mean that she is not the sex she is designated to be, but, rather, the masculine sex *encore* (and *en corps*) parading in the mode of otherness. For Irigaray, that phallogocentric mode of signifying the female sex perpetually reproduces phantasms of its own self-amplifying desire. Instead of a self-limiting linguistic gesture that grants alterity or difference to women, phallogocentrism offers a name to eclipse the feminine and take its place' (12–13).

I would not attempt to represent what 'woman' might be outside this phallogocentrism – there are extensive debates about this among feminist theorists (Moi 2000) – but I would incline to say that it is not confined to what the signifying systems of 'sex' and 'gender' usually represent. It may in fact belong to that alteritous smooth space of our BwO, the 'Body of Reality.' Certainly Deleuze and Guattari imply as much when they imagine that part of becoming different to the territorialized BwO entails 'becoming woman.' This would suggest becoming less phallic. The intertextual ensemble alludes nowhere to the alterity of that reality, but instead to the aggressive insistence of the phallus, which means that it understands both men and women in essentially similar ways. Its phallic representation of women's bodies erases the potential difference that women could bring to physical culture by virtue of their difference. The parergonality of the texts renders second the non-phallic reality of the body.

The phallus symbolizes the desire for sovereignty that emerges from the wider history of patriarchal, European expansionism. Mark Taylor (1984) finds that 'the link between the political and sexual economy of domination is patriarchy.' The phallus signifies that link in the desire to penetrate otherness such that it comes under the authority of the sovereign self. Parallelling Butler's well-trodden explication of gender as a performance that produces the effective illusion of an originary gendered identity, the phallus performs the will to power that produces the illusion of an originary modern sovereign selfhood. The formation of the fit body is a phallic performance that makes our BwO appear to be individual and sovereign. The intertextual ensemble writes the script for this performance. Phallic desire establishes the link between the cosmology of the technology of physical fitness – i.e., the descriptive, hermeneutic structure that makes it intelligible – and the actual production (inscription and prescription) of the life that its hermeneutics describes. The various centrisms (human, ego, and youth) that I said above make sense of the technology of physical fitness come to life in the phallic colonization of our BwO, which is the reproduction of the taught, strong, impermeable, fit, independent body. In short, the cosmology that centres on the sovereignty of human, self, and youth is actualized by phallic desire. While our ensemble does everything that it can to foster this kind of desire – that is what the processes of inscription and prescription set out to accomplish, as I try to show below – ultimately no one 'can keep it up,' and many others do not even want to. Modern death marks the beginning of eternal impotence.

This desire for spatial domination has another side: the desire to be closed to the other. The phallic will to power penetrates the otherness of decay, old age, and death to make it dis-appear. For this disappearing act to be successful, the sovereign self must remain impervious to otherness – i.e, it incorporates otherness without being altered by it – even though it lives perpetually in the shadow of the parergonal otherness of death. I have written elsewhere about this other side of phallic desire, metaphorically, as anal closure – the tight anus that resists entry (Pronger 1999b). It is misogynist desire – fearful of becoming open, of being penetrated by the other. In the name of sovereign self-preservation, phallic desire resists being undermined by the outside that it penetrates. Unlike compassionate emptiness, phallic desire produces its reality by domination, instead of by empathetic submission. Submission is anathema to the domination of the phallus. Phallic desire fears femininity, passivity, impotence, permeability. It dreads the spectre of submitting to the ultimate otherness of the sovereign self, which is its essential lack of sovereignty. This fear of otherness comes from the abjection of alterity, which is nothing less than the loss of the infinitely interdependent reflecting body, the One Bright Pearl, which is the infinity of our BwO, realized by our wave nature, the smooth space of movement. Phallic desire cuts us off from our infinite potential and has us make do with the finite reality of the body that has been territorialized by pouvoir, realized in particle nature, in the alienating, striated space of movement. Loss and lack. The majestic, territorializing performance of the phallus turns out to be quite the opposite: abjecting infinity and grasping at meagre finitude. The fear of being penetrated by alterity makes us smaller. The phallus, in short, is pathetic.

Drawing on the work of ecofeminists, deep ecologists, and Heidegger, Patricia Glazebrook (in press) has written about the ways in which the phallic logic of domination underscores the entire modernist project and is at the core of environmental destruction. I would add that our phallic desire for sovereignty, by cutting us off from the infinity of interdependent reflecting body, the wave nature of our BwO, is the alienating energy that makes it possible for us to wreck the ecosphere as though it were not profoundly part of us as we constitute ourselves in our particle nature. Only by overcoming this phallic alienation from the infinity of the BwO, can we hope to live more harmoniously.

Phallic desire dominates and limits not only its environment, but also the self. There is a tragic irony in the phallic quest for sovereignty, in its perpetual, selfish, domineering erection of youth. The very process of sovereign independence is quite the opposite. The forces of pouvoir territorialize our BwO. The technology of the modern (fit) self (Foucault 1988; Miller 1993) is actually *subjection* in the cosmological disguise of independent sovereignty. The sovereign-seeking phallic self is the *chora* (receptacle) of pouvoir. Imagining itself as fucking the world to take space for itself, the phallic body is actually getting fucked by pouvoir and bearing its children, as it were. In a typically patriarchal fashion, technology fucks the space of the body, occupies and makes it its own, trying to reproduce itself in its own image. In chapter 2, I wrote about the open space of movement and proposed that it is the very opening that makes possible the energy of both pouvoir and puissance. Understood phallically, this is the open space through which the modern technology of resource management and exploitation enters the body. This phallic organization and use of the energy of puissance striate the smooth space of the body, the infinite dimensionality of movement.

To reiterate my thesis so far. The cosmology to which the intertextual ensemble appeals for its intelligibility posits the centrality of human, self, and youth and appeals to the phallic desire to dominate the smooth space of our BwO. This is the paradigm of the body at work in the exercise sciences.[4] I have been suggesting that this is a discursive organization of our BwO, whose parergonality renders second the infinitely interdependent reflecting body (the 'Body of Reality'). And, as Foucault (1981) has written, discourse works by 'the action of an imposed scarcity, with a fundamental power of affirmation' (73). The power of this affirmation depends upon the denial of the fulness of puissance, imposing on its infinite productivity the libidinal economy of lack. It is a productive and dynamic discourse of sovereignty. The quest for sovereignty is its affirmative element. The affirmative assumption that sovereignty needs to be achieved conceals the imposition of its actual scarcity.

The discourse of sovereignty and its libidinal economy of lack, I have argued, constitute the energy source of modern phallic desire. It is the desiring engine of consumption and production, in science, technology, education, commerce, medicine, and physical fitness, among other areas. So modernity frees the body of the tyranny of the inherent codes that was the business of the premodern socius, wherein the codes of 'nature' (good and evil, heavenly and earthly, spirit and body, man and woman, black and white, and so on) limited the production of life. 'To code desire – and the fear, the anguish of decoded flows – is the business of the socius' (Deleuze and Guattari 1987, 139). Freed of the codes of its natures, modern desire is recoded by its value to the myriad projects of sovereignty. The texts of the technology of physical fitness code desire to increase its value to the sovereignty of the body. Yet such a quest for sovereignty is in actuality subjection to the discourse of sovereignty and its presumption of the body's fundamental lack. Bodies operating within the discourse are territorialized by this libidinal economy of lack. The infinite wealth of puissance is thus rendered poor.

Salvation and Accumulation

Representing the body as seriously lacking, facing the abyss of failed sovereign selfhood, the intertextual ensemble implies that the body needs the salvation that the technology of physical fitness affords. It models modern salvation on the accumulative parergonal logic of consumer capitalism, which claims that the solution to lack lies in the accumulation of wealth. For example, those who can afford to do so, plan for the lack that is thought to constitute old age by accumulating capital investments that might soften its misery and reduce the risk of dying early and poor. Consumerism promises that we can find happiness and meaning in life by accumulating property that entertains, shelters, and defines us, building our self-esteem, enabling us both to identify with and to distinguish ourselves from others by the accumulation and display of our consumer tastes (Miles 1998). The power to accumulate is directly related to the power to produce the wealth that purchases consumer products, and so success depends on rational management and exploitation of resources.

Mark Taylor (1987) points out that Heidegger, Bataille, Levinas, and Kierkegaard have criticized the way of life that is geared to productive expenditure of energy in the parergonal logics of profitability and reasonable return on investments. It organizes existence around systems of accounting and accountability:

> 'Reason,' Bataille maintains, 'is bound up with work and the purposive activity that incarnates its laws.' (Bataille 1977, p. 168) Work, in turn is governed by the principle of *utility*. In Hegel's System, reasonable activity is, by definition, purposeful. The worker sees profitable return on every investment of his or her time and energy. When the System is working at maximum efficiency, nothing is useless. The Hegelian economy actually assumes full employment in which no one is *désoeuvré:* out of work, unoccupied or idle. To preserve itself, a utilitarian system must *exclude* what is useless or profitless. Consequently, work is inextricably bound up with a complex network of prohibitions. While reasonable work and the work of reason rest on taboos, taboos work by excluding or repressing that which disrupts productive labour. For Bataille, the two

primary forces interrupting purposive activity are *eros* and *thanatos*. In his consideration of 'the interdependent ensemble of prohibitions,' Bataille stresses that 'for all known peoples, the world of work opposes that of sexuality and death.' (Bataille, nd #1683, p. 33) Inverting the customary association of the sacred with order (cosmos) and the profane with disorder (chaos), Bataille contends that the world of work is profane and the forbidden domain circumscribed by work is sacred. (Taylor 1987, 131)

Work and accounting for work ensure the proper discipline for the productive expenditure of energy that makes consumption possible. For those who live middle-class, 'productive' lives, this certainly is not news. And those who find such a life less than edifying are often aware of the ways in which productivity and profitability depend on the parergonal logic of particular systems of accumulation and accounting. Some things just do not figure into the system, and others are outright prohibited.

The parergonal logic of financial capital accumulation is similarly at work in the intertextual ensemble of the technology of physical fitness, where the body accumulates physical capital within the parameters of physical fitness, in terms of aerobic capacity, strength, flexibility, fat-to-lean ratios, attractiveness, and so on. This capital is accumulated by the productive and disciplined way of life that includes regular exercise and controlled diet. Bataille says that the eclipse of the sacred in the profanity of productive work is a serious degradation of our potential for realization – all the more so, I suggest, when such productivity is directed at the life of the body, at controlling the ways in which it expends its energies, at delimiting its power of connection (puissance).

From Foucault's perspective, the vast disciplinary technology of the modern workplace keeps people working at maximum efficiency. The rewards, of course, are increased power in the economics of production and consumption. But the power that the modern disciplined life gains in economic utility it loses in political and ontological agency. For Foucault (1979), the body is at the very heart of this phenomenon. He comments on the advent of the body politics of modern discipline in the eighteenth century:

The historical moment of the disciplines was the moment when an art of the body was born, which was directed not only at the growth of its skills, nor at the intensification of its subjection, but at the formation of a relation that in the mechanism itself makes it more obedient as it becomes more useful, and conversely. What was then being formed was a policy of coercions that act upon the body, a calculated manipulation of its elements, its gestures, its behaviour. The human body was entering a machinery of power that explores it, breaks it down and rearranges it. A 'political anatomy', which was also a 'mechanics of power', was being born; it defined how one may have a hold over others' bodies, not only so that they may do what one wishes, but so that they may operate as one wishes, with the techniques, the speed and the efficiency that one determines. Thus discipline produces subjected and practised bodies, 'docile bodies.' Discipline increases the forces of the body (in economic terms of utility) and diminishes these same forces (in political terms of obedience). In short it dissociates power [puissance] from the body; on the one hand, it turns it into an 'aptitude', a 'capacity', which it seeks to increase [in our case, the physical fitness of the body, its 'sovereignty']; on the other hand, it reverses the course of the energy, the power that might result from it, and turns it into a relation of strict subjection. If economic exploitation separates the force and the product of labour, let us say that disciplinary coercion establishes in the body the constricting link between an increased aptitude and an increased domination. (138)

The technology of physical fitness also works within this profane framework of productive expenditure that increases aptitude by increasing domination. It promises that the more productively the body is trained, the more thoroughly it is called to account for itself, and the more able-bodied it becomes, the more it will increase its power to purchase modern sovereign self-hood. The central rite of the technology is exercise, commonly called a 'workout.' And its soteriological promise is the same as the famous words over the gates of the Auschwitz concentration camp: 'Arbeit macht Frei' '(Work shall make you free).' Modern salvation comes from work, which promises to purchase freedom. How this functions in physical fitness we see in the next sub-sections on inscription and prescription.

My final point in this section on the description of the body is that the cosmology of the sovereignty of humanity, has a soteriology that operates on the logic that individuals can accumulate the 'freedom' of sovereignty by accumulating capital from individual work, not by receiving grace. Salvation comes from individual self's working. Only the epidemiological texts of health promotion conceptualize salvation beyond the individual, calculating the cost–benefit ratios of an exercising and diet-conscious population. These are what Foucault called the biopolitics of the population, which goes to work in the anatamo-politics of the individual. As I said above, health promotion deals with the population's health, but its solution is to target the individual. Foucault (1979) puts it this way: 'It [is] a question not of treating the body, *en masse*, as if it were an indisociable unity [our BwO, perhaps], but of working it "retail", individually; of exercising upon it a subtle coercion, of obtaining holds upon it at the level of the mechanism itself – movements, gestures, attitudes, rapidity: an infinitesimal power over the *active body*' (137, emphasis added). And it is the work of inscription and prescription to take this 'hold' over the active body.

The pernicious twist in this modern technological soteriology is that the promise of freedom is not freedom at all, but individuals' subjection to the reterritorializing power of pouvoir, to live a limited and aggressively technological life, re-sourced by pouvoir. Salvation by *self*-sovereignty defeats itself. The logic of mastery that was part of the construction of God/man, which modernity inverts as the self-mastery of man, is actually the mastery of Gestell as an overwhelming cultural force. The technology of physical fitness could be said to recast Luther's famous soteriological claim of 'salvation by faith alone' as 'salvation by work alone.' As we see below, for the fitness-bound body this work takes a great deal of discipline, in Foucault's sense. This modernist soteriology is thus problematic not only for the way in which it constructs the self, but also in how it serves the larger processes of modernity, making humans into resources by territorializing their desire.

This disciplinary anatamo-politics of the body, which is the microlevel at which individuals commit themselves to the biopolitical, technological project of pouvoir, requires faith in the soteriological power of technology. And that power consists of its ability to turn what simply is in its own right (including the body) into what is for us humans. *Pro nobis* and *pro me*: a soteriology that is as at least as old as the Book of Genesis and finds its personal intensification in Luther's individualized soteriology. Faith in technology depends on belief in the rightness of directing our consciousness and actions *pro nobis* and *pro me*. And the technological spin on this is faith in the power (pouvoir) of domination, which can force things to be *pro nobis* and *pro me*. Thus faith in the technology of physical fitness depends on a commitment to domination as a founding way of life. By embracing that faith, individuals open themselves to the biopolitical project of pouvoir. And just as anxiety about the salvation of the soul worked as the point of access for an earlier Christian 'evangelism of fear' (Delumeau 1990, 112–13), so too, as Baudrillard has noted, 'the body as a space of desire has become an object of salvation, which has in its ideological functions replaced the soul' (Bell 1985, 37).

Michelle Lelwica (1999) says that 'religion refers to cultural systems of meaning consisting of rituals, symbols, stories, and beliefs, whose special task is to present a picture of the whole of life in relation to which human experiences become meaningful. Religions provide idioms for articulating what is most important in life, a task that becomes especially important in times of suffering and confusion.' The technology of physical fitness calls on the cosmology of modern humanism. Articulating the modernist belief in the ultimate importance of humanity, self, phallus, and youth, it tells a story of the body. It promises some salvation from the suffering and confusion of old age and death by the soteriological power of physical work, demanding the disciplined rituals of exercise and dietary vigilance. The technology of physical fitness is in fact therefore a religious approach to the body. And like its patriarchal Christian predecessor, it reproduces itself by exploiting human vulnerability and promulgating a culture of fear.

'Salvation' comes from subjecting the body to the parergonality of sovereignty, centred on humanism, egocentrism, youth-centrism, and phallocentrism. It is subjection in that it denies that which is other to these centrisms – specifically, the infinite multiplicity of the BwO, which is reflected, for example, in the myth of Indra's Net. While this cosmology, and its phallic will-to-the-power-of-subjection, have many adherents and proponents – the writers and enthusiastic readers of the intertextual ensemble in particular – there are many people who are not so easily enticed and who find it difficult or even undesirable to follow the path of salvation that the cosmology describes. This could explain why, even though it is widely believed that discipline in diet and physical activity will save people from numbers of diseases, and delay death, the vast majority of people do not follow such discipline (Katzmarzyk, Gledhill, and Shephard 2000). The processes of inscription and prescription attempt to draw people into the soteriology, to make the puissant energy of the BwO available to the modernist imperative for resource development – pouvoir.

Inscription

Bruno Latour studied the production of scientific knowledge in the laboratory. He focused on the way in which the production of texts makes scientific knowledge and on how that production is a social enterprise (Latour and Woolgar 1986). My analysis mirrors Latour's in so far as it also looks at the construction of techno-scientific facts about the body as a social phenomenon that takes place in the production of texts. But whereas research science produces texts about reality *in general*, the technology of physical fitness produces texts about *individual* bodies on the basis of general knowledge constructed in the laboratory. As Rouse (1987) has shown, laboratory life is reproduced outside the laboratory in the everyday world: 'Developments become disseminated into the world outside the laboratory by standardizing scientific techniques and equipment and by adjusting nonscientific practices and situations to make them amenable to the employment of scientific materials and practices. The result is that the world is increasingly a made world, in the sense that it reflects the systematic extension of ... technical capacities, the equipment they employ, and the phenomena they make manifest' (211).

In what follows in this chapter I attempt to show how the socially constructed world of the exercise science laboratory – its technological approach to the body – is represented in everyday life through the textual production of physical fitness testing and other elements of the intertextual ensemble. This then is an account of the ways in which the texts of the technology of physical fitness 'make people up' (Hacking 1992; 1995).

The cosmology and soteriology described above form the hermeneutic context for understanding the body as a technological project, a resource that needs to be managed in order to be saved from the abjection from which it suffers within that cosmology. The cosmology makes puissance available to pouvoir. In the techno-culture of physical fitness, this project appears textually through various processes of inscription and prescription, which produce a logocentric simulacrum of the modernist cosmology and soteriology of the body in the puissance of the actual living, moving body.

The technology of physical fitness consists not simply of the detached, theoretical musings of government officials and research scientists, or the concepts of popular writers on fitness, manufacturers of fitness products, and the media. As we see in this section, it territorializes the BwO. First, it inscribes individual bodies with the codes of the technology, using concentric circles of texts that delimit the paradigm; techniques of personal accountability, including confession; and rhetorics of authority and exclusion that further isolate the faithful. Second, it prescribes a technological production of desire in which participants write their own narrative and pursue salvation through consumption of physical fitness.

Circles of Texts

Inscription and prescription are practices that constitute the organizational gaze, as Foucault (1975) would say, of the modern technological production of the body. The whole point of the intertextual ensemble is to produce modern technological desire on the BwO. As Rouse would say of the texts of science, they too are engaged profoundly with the production of reality – applied texts, in every sense. Their intertextuality is important, for together they knit a technological culture of the body as it can be realized by fitness technologies. More specifically, they inscribe the body in a fourfold circle of texts: interactive texts, direct reference texts, ambient texts, and shadow texts. Together these produce a discourse on the body through which it can be read and by which its future can be charted.

First, interactive texts directly address individuals and are produced as a result of that address. The Canadian ministry of health, for example, has produced a *Physical Activity Guide* that speaks to the reader directly: 'Improving *your* health through physical activity is easier than *you* think' (Health Canada, n.d., 2, emphasis added). Scientific fitness testing, popular fitness manuals and log books, and exercise equipment such as heart rate monitors also address readers directly, producing texts on the specific bodies of the people who read them. In a fitness test, for instance, the procedures of the test themselves are textual, because they treat the body as an object that produces signs that can be measured and calculated, or *read* and inscribed, through the logos of the procedures. The procedures of a fitness test compel the body to move in very precise ways so that it can be read in the language of the science of physical fitness, making the body appear in much the same way it does inside the laboratory. This is an example of the 'tight coupling' between laboratory and day-to-day life that Rouse has said characterizes scientifically produced society. So the texts of the test include procedures followed, tasks performed, data entry, computer printouts, and 'behaviour reinforcement tools' (Canadian Association of Sport Sciences 1987) and other printed 'inspirational' tracts that teach participants how to read their own bodies according to the paradigms of the test, the science, and modern technoculture. And all these are read back into the body, which becomes the primary text. In a more complex way, popular representations of the fit body produce interactive texts, in so far as people read them in comparison with themselves and in the context of their desires – in effect reading themselves within the iconography of the fit body.

Because of their interactivity, the first circle of texts is dynamic. I place these texts first because they try to make life conform to the world and cosmology of the technological paradigm – they are 'frontline' texts that disseminate the reality and productive knowledge of the exercise science laboratory into the rest of the world,[5] and they bring macro-systemic discourses of the body to bear upon the microsystems of individuals. As interventions into the lives of people, they are constitutive in that they attempt actually to make people up (Hacking 1992), giving them a particular kind of knowledge of the body, attempting to motivate them to move, to produce their desires in certain ways. The other circles of texts background this interpellation.

Also among the first circle of texts we find 'lifestyle questionnaires,' such as the 'Computerized Lifestyle Assessment' (Skinner 1994a). It employs a battery of modified scientific questionnaires that are used for assessing people's 'health status' (for example, the *Alcohol Dependency Scale* and the *Drug Abuse Screening Test*, which Skinner (1994b, 32) says studies have shown to be highly effective in producing accurate DSM-III diagnosis). The questionnaires interrogate and assess the following personal 'lifestyle areas': nutrition, eating habits, caffeine use, physical activity, body weight, sleep, social relationships, family interactions, tobacco use, alcohol use, non-medical drug use, medical/ dental care, motor vehicle safety, sexual activities, work and leisure, and emotional health. The authors of the test claim that it is instrumental, for instance, in directing people who are not sufficiently physically active to submit to physical fitness testing, counselling, and exercise prescription (Skinner 1994b). In this way it attempts to inject into the lives of individuals links to other interactive texts.

Other popular interactive texts are on-line personal assessment tools such as those offered at Asimba, a fitness-oriented product-marketing website that describes itself as 'the authentic community for all *your* active lifestyle needs, and the catalyst to improve the quality of life through fitness, sports, nutrition' (http://www.asimba.com/asm/ Home, emphasis added). Asimba offers a variety of appraisal devices such as the 'Body Mass Index,' the 'Burn Calculator' (which calculates the number of calories an individual will burn in given physical activities), 'Resting Metabolic Rate Calculator,' and electronic log books for training.

Fitness for Dummies™ (Schlosberg and Neporent 1996) encourages readers to go to a fitness club and get a fully-fledged fitness test done by accredited fitness appraisers. It also describes less formal and less accurate tests that readers can do to inscribe their bodies in terms of aerobic fitness, fatness, and body strength. Fitness magazines regularly offer questionnaires and physical assessment techniques as well. And the assessments usually recommend that readers keep a record of their assessments in order to read future assessment texts against past. Fitness products and services also write interactive texts on individual bodies. The most common of such inscribing products is probably the home bathroom scale, the more sophisticated of which come with the capacity to measure fat content, as in the 'Tanita Body Fat Monitor.' Computerized aerobic training machines such as stair climbers, treadmills, stationary bicycles, and rowing ergometers produce electronic texts that inscribe the number of calories being burned, as well as charting heart rate. More advanced machines 'interface' with computers that inscribe power output over time.

As I pointed out above, some of the products allow users to download the inscriptions to personal computers in order to produce an ongoing narrative on the individual's physical, and in some cases emotional, development. Training log books are interactive inscribing devices. Personal trainers inscribe the bodies of their clients, as well, often keeping written records of their clients' bodies and way of life. An advertisement for a fitness club in Toronto, called 'Fitness One on One,' has a picture of a serious-looking, muscular young man, with his arms crossed, staring straight at the reader; the ad copy says: 'He knows where you live; he knows what you eat; he knows what you did last weekend; and you're going to thank him for it' (*Toronto Life*, January 2000, 112). Personal trainers' speech acts, in which they give off-the-cuff assessments of the bodies of their clients, are interactive inscribing practices, which may or may not turn out to be ephemeral, depending on the memories of the trainers and clients. In my experience, such casual assessments have been inscribed in my memory for a long time; some had powerful effects on how I read my body and on how I exercised my desire.

The second circle of texts consists of those that are directly referenced in the first, giving background support to them. In some cases this is a scholarly referencing system. For instance, the procedural manual for the Canadian Standardized Test of Fitness (CSTF) refers to forty-three publications: ten are institutional reports; twenty-seven are from scholarly journals in medical and exercise physiology; four are from exercise physiology textbooks, one is a popular book of behavioural science (Davis, Fanning, and McKay 1983), and one is from a professional journal (the *Canadian Association for Health, Physical Education and Recreation Journal*). The CSTF's *Interpretation and Counselling Manual* also offers thirty-three 'Suggested Reading[s]' for 'professionals' (i.e., certified fitness appraisers) and 'clients.' It advises professionals to read exercise physiology texts such as the *American College of Sports Medicine's Resource Guidelines for Exercise Testing and Prescription* (ACSM 1993), manuals on 'counselling and communications skills' such as *The Skilled Helper* (Egan 1975), as well as government documents on 'fitness and lifestyle' such as Fitness Ontario's *Sticking with Fitness* (Fitness Ontario 1984), which 'provides an update summary of research on *adherence* and practical implications for fitness leaders' (Canadian Association of Sport Sciences 1987a, 42, emphasis added). 'Clients' of the fitness test are advised to read books such as *The Aerobics Program for Total Well-Being* (Cooper 1982), *Eating for the Health of It: A New Look at Nutrition* (MacDonald 1985), or various pamphlets available through government agencies (such as Participaction and Fitness Canada), life insurance companies (such as Metropolitan Life), food manufacturers (such as Kellogg's), and medical associations (such as the Canadian Heart and Stroke Foundation).

While most popular texts and fitness products do not engage in the rigorous and exclusive referencing of authoritative institutional science, they frequently do refer to such authority by oblique references to what 'science' or 'experts' say, which for many readers is probably sufficient rhetorically. Some publications in the popular fields, however, do appeal to scientific authority by referencing institutional science. Bill Phillips's *Sport Supplement Review* (1997), for instance, lists 304 items, almost all of which are from 'legitimate' peer-reviewed scientific publishing. Each of the sixteen chapters of *The Triathlete's Training Bible* lists on average twenty-five references from academic science publishing (Friel 1998). While *Fitness for Dummies*™ (Schlosberg and Neporent 1996) does not offer academic references, co-author Liz Neporent has a master of science degree in exercise physiology, as well as certifications with the ACSM and the (U.S.) National Strength and Conditioning Association. While these popular texts are not as rigorous as the academic texts in their scholarly invocation of the second circle, they are, as I hope to show, just as rigorous in their cultural invocation, indeed reproduction, of modern technological cosmology and soteriology.

The third circle of texts is ambient. Not directly mentioned in the first circle, these texts nevertheless contribute to its context, intelligibility, and authority. Ambient texts support the inscribing work of the first two circles by enhancing their cultural credibility. In this way they are different from the fourth circle – to which the first two also do not directly refer – which lies in the shadow of the technological project. The tightest ambient texts come from academic science: these are the texts to which the second circle of (referenced) texts refer, as well as the myriad regression of texts referenced there – every scholarly text cited in third-circle texts refers to more scholarly texts, which in turn refer to more scholarly texts, which refer to more scholarly texts, and so on (see chapter 1 above). As both Latour and Bazerman have argued, scientific texts are primarily constructed out of the other texts to which they refer. The scientific culture of referencing is highly exclusive. So, for instance, the only texts referenced in the CSEP's fitness test are those with 'official' status – i.e., texts produced under the authority of credentiallized science or endorsed by that science. Third-circle texts are 'legitimately' referenced in the first two circles under that authority. This is not to say that all them are scholarly science; however, they become part of the circle by virtue of the combined authority of the scientific and institutional realms of discourse – in this case, the CSEP and the government of Canada. This authority comes from thirty years of political manoeuvring in university physical education, through which the biophysical sciences have come to dominate knowledge production (MacIntosh 1986). That is the 'technicist tendency' in physical education, a technological orientation to knowledge and to life standard now in many other academic fields, especially in the health sciences. The unifying feature of these ambient texts is their commitment to the cosmological paradigm of the technology of physical fitness and their exclusion of others paradigms and possibilities.[6]

More complex ambient texts also contribute to the background of the first two circles but are not part of the formal culture of science. Less rigorously policed by peer review and other techniques of academic control, they are nevertheless influential and often uncompromising in their representation of how the body ought to be. These are the more obliquely referenced texts on the body that circulate in consumer culture more generally. Pre-eminent among them are those omnipresent texts of advertising that represent various versions of the slim, muscular, and physically fit body. They also include the texts of television and film that feature such bodies. Packaging of consumer goods represents such bodies – for example, the packaging that surrounds a pair of Calvin Klein underpants, which always features partially clad bodies. Representations of the fit body in pornography contribute to the ambience. And even more oblique, but perhaps more powerful, are the unwritten texts about body shape that circulate in the day-to-day interactions of people, judging and speaking about the attractiveness and acceptability of different kinds of bodies. As numbers of scholars have argued, magazines, advertisements, television, packaging, and film also represent discourses about what kinds of bodies embody model citizenship in terms of health, productivity, and self-responsibility (Bordo 1993; Robert Crawford 1984; Trish Crawford 1995; Featherstone 1991; Miller 1993) and spiritual development (Lelwica 1999).

And, despite some variety in the look of the bodies represented in this non-scientific third circle of texts, like the scientific texts they support each other and the first two circles in their assumption of the cosmological paradigm of modern humanity – an assumption that is very influential in the Zeitgeist of modern culture, both popular and elite. The most extensive critical work on the power of these popular representations has been done by feminist scholars critiquing the power of the images of slim women. Many observers have argued that these representations have been so powerful that many women find it difficult to think outside them. While there certainly are gendered dimensions to that imagery, the power of popular body images, especially in their technological dimension, is not only gendered and is not limited to women and girls.

The exclusionary power of the first three circles of texts forms a fourth, which I call the circle of 'shadow texts.' These are other textual discourses on the body that belong in neither the popular nor the scientific canon on the fit body. Some are part of the academy but shadowed by the exercise sciences – for instance, the literature on the phenomenology of the body in philosophy, existential psychology, nursing, and education. Alternative accounts of health, the body, and fitness in feminist writing have marginal or no presence in the inner circles. Non-modern, non-Western ethno-cultural traditions also have produced very different texts on health and the ontology of the body. There are critical textual discourses on the body, such as queer theory and continental European philosophy, whose voice is for the most part silent in the intertextual ensemble. Yet another realm of shadowed texts contains individuals' own experiences, knowledge, or narratives on the body.[7]

And the texts most powerfully shadowed are those that write against the modernist project and cosmology, which invite readers to move beyond texts and modern cosmology. Certainly among these is a rich history of religious texts that suggest the body's potential to live beyond its inscriptions: Tantra, Yoga, Zen, Kabala, Sufism, and Christian mysticisms, to mention only a few. Nothing of these shadow discourses appears anywhere in the first three circles of texts. Yoga and the Eastern martial arts do figure in the cult of physical fitness, as any trip to the self-help section of a bookstore will show. But they do not participate in the discourse for their *transcendental* potential – although for some readers that may well be their ultimate effect. Within the cult of physical fitness they are legitimate for the way in which they contribute to the resourcing of human potential in the technological project. The fact that these, and other physical fitness practices, may also portend powers that transcend the technological project is important and, as I argue in my Postscript, offers some reason for hope. My argument here is that the circle of texts does not foster that potential – quite the opposite.

The outer (fourth) circle constitutes the boundary that attempts to separate out all that is not part of the modern technological cosmos. It is a complex and contested project that tries to make the space of the body purely modern. The contest takes place in conflicts over what texts become available to readers of the body. On a variety of other fronts, this has been the struggle of feminists, anti-racists, gay and lesbian liberationists, queer activists, and postmodern critics of the dominance of patriarchal, racist, heterosexist, normative, modernist narratives of the body. I am highlighting it similarly viz-à-vis the hegemonic texts of physical fitness. The exclusion of these shadow discourses forms a crucial element in the rhetoric of the first three circles of texts, which together attempt to produce a resourceful government of the body.

The four circles of texts centre on the modern individual subject that I described above in this chapter. They circle in on the infinite surface of BwO, inscribing finite, modern, fit or unfit, technological subjects, calling the body to account for itself as such. I use the metaphor of the circle to suggest the way in which reality is produced when it is encircled. When a hunting party encircles a fox, the animal ceases to be just a fox in the woods, going about its own business; it becomes prey. Similarly, when one comes to read oneself through the interactive texts, one is encircled by the layers and exclusions of the circle of texts and is pressed to become what the texts inscribe. The circle of texts addresses the individual, which is already a territorialization of the BwO. Approached as an individual, one (i.e., the territorialized BwO) is likely to respond as one. The fox hunted as prey responds as prey.

But whereas foxes invariably try to escape being prey, most modern humans do not seem to try to escape their individuality. Encircled by these layers of texts, they find it difficult to see beyond them, to reach the infinite reality that lies beyond the perimeter of the fourth circular boundary. It is not impossible. But the circularity of the texts offers the reader no help in seeing beyond – quite the opposite. As Glass would say, the circle highlights our particle nature and obscures our wave nature. Here is the most important problem posed by the encircling texts: they foster no alterity from themselves. They do not have complete authority over the ontology of the reader/read; skilled readers can extricate themselves from the circle. But the rhetorical structure of this layering of texts is geared not to facilitating escape from the modern technological project, but rather to coercing submission to it by circumscribing puissance in concentric layers of text. For the philosophy of the limit, the circles of texts form a parergonal logic for reading the body, systematically producing and reinforcing one reading of the body that renders second others, foreclosing on alterity. It is a textual type of bullying.

The encircling texts of the ensemble provoke the body to appear in a certain way and then represent that appearance in a process of inscription and calculation, interpreting and consequently prescribing a way of life based on the representation. What kind of body, what kind of desire, is made to appear in such a process of provocation, inscription, calculation, interpretation, and prescription? How do these science-based texts interpellate or hail the body, as Althuser would say (1977)? How does this textual process govern desire?

The interactive texts of the technology of physical fitness directly address individual bodies, calling them to account according to their resource value for the sovereign project. Various systems that evaluate their physical capital make these bodies accountable. Evaluative codes mark the body's accumulation of physical capital that will afford it sovereign power, both in its ability to function in the present and as a calculation of its vulnerability in the future. The body is coded in exercise protocols according to frequency, intensity, time, and type of movement (which the exercise sciences call the FITT principle). The more popular textual fields also code the body – less scientifically but just as technologically – for its accumulation of capital in terms of symbolic exchange value: the relative value of different body shapes in terms of attractiveness, youthfulness, masculinity, femininity, whiteness, slimness, muscularity, able-bodiedness, and normality. This kind of physical capital affords its owners greater or lesser self-esteem (which is clearly part of the sovereign project) and purchases the potential for sexual experience, respectability, and status, promising to fill the void (Lelwica 1999) that the modernist discourse of lack inscribes. The standards of such evaluations are constantly changing and reflect the fashions of popular representations of the body that circulate in the media and in the daily interactions of people. There are also different standards of the body according to differences of gender, race, class, (dis)ability, and sexuality. What all the evaluative systems, both scientific and popular, and standards have in common, however, is the paradigmatic assumption that the body's values can be increased by its technological development, by cultivating it as a resource. But this takes some convincing, which is the role inscription.

Accounting for Oneself

The BwO is inscribed with its functional use-values as an organism, which is a codification of the body's value as 'physical capital' (Bourdieu 1988; Shilling 1993). This is a matter of discerning the discrete forms of physical capital (for example, the components of fitness, conformity to fashions of body shape) and calculating their value. The point is to assess value and thereby to develop rational action programs (through exercise, diet, and so on) which will accumulate more physical capital. The implicit imperative is for the individual to seek personal profit from the development of his or her body as a capital resource – extracting as much value from it as possible. Abstract values are routinely assigned to resources: in the case of finance capital, value is monetary (dollars, for example); in the case of physical fitness capital, scientific value is expressed as VO_2max. $(ml/kg^{-1}/min^{-1})$, body mass index (kg/m^2), grip strength (kg), and so on. Where value can be established, there is the potential for increased value. A profit motive is invoked here. The body is understood not in terms of its capacity for puissant intensity, but in terms of capital growth. The less capital the body holds, the less potential it has; conversely, increased capital leads to greater potential. This is the soteriology of consumption: the more capital one accumulates, the more one can afford to save oneself by consuming. Functional capacities (aerobic capacity, strength, flexibility, youthfulness, slenderness, muscularity, and so on), coded for their capital use-value, can purchase salvation.

This is a business model of salvation: improving the efficiency and output of the organization/organism will increase profitability and save one from going under. For example, an increased capacity to metabolize fats, a high energy source, is the result of a combination of three factors – better cardiovascular function, which results from a rational program of aerobic exercise; greater muscle mass, which can follow from a program of resistance training; and a decreased ratio of fat to lean in body composition, which results from a combination of caloric restraint in diet, more aerobic activity, and increased muscle mass (which increases metabolism). Increased power can result from stronger muscles, which allow one to do more work as a result of resistance strength training. The efficient extraction and development of the body's puissance as an energy resource can increase the body's physical capital. This power and efficiency keep the organism fit, thus maintaining or even improving its position in the marketplace of sovereignty.

'Capital resource development' gives a modern twist to a very old soteriological narrative form. The story of St Paul is perhaps the original inspiration for this twisted modern narrative: a sinner experiences the light of truth and is saved from the abyss. But the soteriological power derived from the technology of physical fitness is unlike the salvation of Paul, who, according to the Bible, 'saw the light' on the road to Damascus and was saved by the 'Grace of God' – an unmerited gift that inspired him to devote himself to his fellow human beings in the development of emergent communities (the early churches) that challenged dominant (Greek, Roman, and Hebrew) paradigms for the meaning of life. Salvation by the technology of physical fitness has nothing to do with emergent communities developing counterhegemonic paradigms for the meaning of life inspired by the freedom of anything even remotely resembling 'divine grace' but is entirely dependent on the individual's earning salvation for himself or herself, alone, in accordance with the dominant paradigms of modern technology, capital accumulation, and consumption. It is a story of individual salvation by selfish technological 'good works' of accumulation. Here is a dark promise of salvation by subordination to the dominating spirit of pouvoir, the resourcing of the essence of human being in the modern, individualizing, captializing biopolitical project. The result is bodies that are increasingly resourced – appreciated not for the way in which they reflect infinity, but for how they grasp at their own sovereignty, a project doomed to failure.

The narrative structure of this discourse is one of closure, the point being to territorialize the openness of the BwO by constructing evaluative 'truths' about particular bodies. As Foucault (1980a) has argued, one of the great techniques for producing such truth is confession: 'The confession became one of the West's most highly valued techniques for producing truth. We have become a singularly confessing society. The confession has spread its effects far and wide. It plays a part in justice, medicine, education, family relationships, and love relations, in the most ordinary affairs of everyday life, and in the most solemn rites; one confesses one's crimes, one's sins, one's thoughts and desires, one's illnesses and troubles' (59).

The confession produces a power relation that serves the inscribing process. Historically, in the Christian Catholic traditions, such power belonged to the church and to its capacity to identify the nature of sin, to hear confession, and to grant absolution to believers so as to clear their consciences of their perceptions of wrongdoing. A moralizing Christian belief system that looks for sin everywhere, and believes it impossible for lowly humans to escape sin, requires some way to reassure the faithful that their sin is not so great, their debt so grossly accumulated over many years of sinful life, that they are inclined to give up the entire Christian enterprise and accept sin as unavoidable and unredeemable. Confession serves the dual function of giving penitents psychic relief from the weight of their waywardness and keeping, indeed constructing, them within the belief system of the church. This same form was later taken up by a more modern belief system: psychiatry. Here absolution comes not from God through the church and its ministers, but from the act of speaking: the patient is encouraged to face his or her problematic (neurotic) self and, with the guidance of the psychoanalyst, to attain a cure for his or her neurosis – the famous 'talking cure' (Deleuze and Guattari 1983, 34ff).

Similarly, the intertextual ensemble of the technology of physical fitness encourages readers to confess. Confessional techniques abound in its interactive texts, such as fitness appraisals and log books where participant-readers record what they eat, the intensity, type, and duration of their exercise, and their feelings. Weigh-scales and computerized exercise equipment record the body's confession, unmediated by the consciousness of the person who confesses. The evaluations we make when we look in the mirror and compare our bodies to the popular images of the fit body work as a kind of private confession. And whether we want to or not, we all confess publicly when we remove our clothes in the locker room, at the beach, or in the bedroom.

The form of confession in the first order of texts participates in the process of reterritorialization that Deleuze and Guattari (1983) say is characteristic of the capitalistic tendency to borrow old forms for the recoding of desire: 'Capitalism institutes or restores all sorts of residual and artificial, imaginary, or symbolic territorialisations, thereby attempting, as best it can, to recode, to rechannel persons who have been defined in terms of abstract quantities' (34–5).

The Christian and psychiatric confessional precedents of the intertextual ensemble relied entirely on a speaking subject, who has some power to determine what texts emerge in the act of confession. Of course the church developed powerful tools to get the sinner to confess, such as the promulgation of stigmatic guilt, threats of eternal damnation, and, during the Inquisition, the use of torture. And psychiatry was able to plumb the depths of the unconscious by quite sophisticated techniques of depth analysis, association, hypnotism, and other methods. Nevertheless, the subject retained some power over what 'truths' might appear in his or her words, even if only by stubborn resistance to the process itself. Burnt at the stake, Joan of Arc never confessed, for instance. Fitness testing and other technologies of body monitoring, in contrast, are more effective in extracting confession than their more brutal-seeming predecessors. They remove subjectivity from the body and make it confess as a passive object.[8] Fitness

testing, weigh-scales, and computerized exercise equipment circum-
vent any filtering of the 'truth' through a subject's power of speech,
robbing it of voice, and go right to the body disciplined as an object,
devoid of any power of self-expression and forced to reveal itself in
the codes of exercise science (estimated VO_2max., body mass index,
and so on).

Going right to the disciplined and objectified body, fitness appraisal,
in both its scientific and its more casual mirror comparison forms,
extracts signs of a wayward life: not enough exercise, the wrong kind
of exercise, unhealthy eating habits. And these are moral signs, for the
person who has more physical capital has led a better life, and he or
she who has less of the same is in greater need of salvation. The fitness
test extracts this confession and then, by attempting conversion and a
map for the new life, charts the course for salvation. In Christian
confession, absolution is immediate and unconditional, a simple act of
faith. In psychoanalysis, the cure is slow, but therapeutic techniques
are supposed to free the patient of his or her neuroses, so that he or
she can leave them behind. The reader of fitness texts, however, must
spend the rest of his or her life seeking a cure, which is at best condi-
tional and, in the end, doomed to failure.

Extracting a confession from the body-as-object, unmediated by the
body-as-subject, is a powerful form of closure. Fitness testing forces
the 'truth' of life, the essence of desire as puissance, out of the body,
into a computer, and onto computer printouts. In the interpretation
stage, the appraiser attempts to get the participant-reader to accept
(conversion) the truth that the body has confessed and face the consequences of his or her former way of life, the problems of his or her
desire, and the failure to accumulate sufficient physical capital in the
body.

Foucault (1980a) says: 'The obligation to confess is now relayed
through so many different points, is so deeply ingrained in us, that we
no longer perceive it as the effect of a power that constrains us
[pouvoir]; on the contrary, it seems to us that truth, lodged in our
most secret nature, "demands" only to surface' (60). The most important aspect of the fitness confessional is the way in which it takes the
body/desire and turns it into a field of visibility, open for examination, control, monitoring. Visibility makes pouvoir accessible to puissance. Confession draws out of invisibility the secrets of desire: the
love of sloth, the erotic indulgence of eating 'fattening foods,' the
pleasures of drinking alcohol, using drugs, smoking.

Scientific fitness tests are particularly assiduous in the degree of control that they exert over their subjects, treating them with much the same dominance as the subjects of a scientific experiment, compelling them to follow very specific protocols. In the more popular texts, the readers have more freedom to move in and out of the protocol. For instance, people logged on to a fitness website that provides questionnaires can more easily log off when they don't feel like confessing than can someone in the midst of a fitness test simply stop – although they do have the right to do so even there. Nevertheless, the questionnaires used in websites and published in fitness and lifestyle magazines and in various exercise manuals attempt to elicit confessions from the readers so that their bodies can be evaluated for their fat-to-lean ratios (usually by the body mass index) or for their frequency, intensity, and type of exercise. Popular manuals ask readers to rate themselves against norms for ability to touch their toes, for instance. Confessing to eating is very popular in these texts, and there are myriad calorie calculators and log books through which readers inscribe their confessions. The 'Vivonic Fitness Planner' computer program, for example, downloads to palm-top computers that allow their owners to input data on their eating, drinking, sleeping, and exercising. The Vivonic web page says that one of the great advantages of the system is that it is portable, which allows the owner to take it to the gym, to restaurants, and even to the grocery store in order constantly to keep track of (i.e., confess) their lives (http://www.vivonic.com). As I already mentioned above, computerized fitness machines track the work, in terms of calories burned, for instance, making the body confess in much the same way as in fitness testing. The confessional technology that goes to work in the popular displays of the body is often less explicitly inscribing as these other techniques. There the confessional booth is probably the mirror in which one sees oneself and compares oneself to the widely circulating icons of the fit body. In these comparisons, confession can be as intimate as the feel of flesh jiggling when one moves, a testimony to the failure to be as smooth and hard as the bodies in the magazines and advertisements.

Rhetorics of Authority and Exclusion

The rituals of fitness confession such as fitness testing claim the power to reveal the truth of the body by appealing to the authority of science. The ritual depends on the authority of science to reveal truth. The

CPAFLA manuals, for example, actively invoke the credentials of those who have written them, as part of their ploy for believability. But as I argued above in the theory of science, *'ethos'* is not sufficient for persuasion in science. 'Seeing is believing.' In order to accept a claim in science one must have an empirical experience of the event in which the truth was revealed. In research science, this empirical experience became textually mediated, in the form of journals, since not everyone could be at the experimental event in order to see. Because what is seen in an event is highly debatable, part of scientific truth-claiming is controlling debate so that there can be agreement. *Controlling* debate lies at the heart of research scientific textuality. With the development of scientific writing, in order to control debate, and thus to ensure consensus on the nature of reality that is produced in scientific research, and thus to ensure the continued credibility of science, a host of controlling techniques emerged. But the credibility of science lies in the apparent openness of its epistemology: scientific claims are credible only because people believe that they have the freedom to disagree with scientific representations. The freedom to disagree, a democratic epistemology, is at the core of faith in scientific texts. Where that freedom is curtailed, by less than explicitly visible structures of textual control, faith in the texts is secured under false pretenses. Scientific writing hides its textual control under the guise of simply representing nature as it appeared in the experiment. Scientific texts therefore co-opt consent in bad faith – because the textual environment is so tightly controlled, the actual freedom for dissent is very small. The same controlling techniques, and thus bad faith, I suggest, are operative in fitness testing and other scientific inscriptions of the body, such as weight, body fat, and heart rate monitors.

Believing in the truth claims of fitness's inscribing technologies, such as a fitness test or a body fat monitor, is structurally much the same as believing in the truth claims of research science. In both, procedures take place, results are recorded, and an interpretation of the results is given. Both produce texts in this process. Both attempt to secure the reader's agreement on the truthfulness of the texts' claims on the presumption that the process that produced the claims was transparent – that is, the results and interpretation were simple, socio-culturally unfettered representations of the 'natural' reality that emerged in the procedure. Yet in both cases the textual discourse is so tightly controlled, and so powerfully produced (in Foucault's sense), that simple and unfettered representation of 'reality' is impossible. Moreover, in the case of fitness testing, unfettered representation could well be counterproductive to the aim of the whole enterprise, which is not freely to represent reality(ies), but to change values and behaviour. Both the texts of research science and fitness's inscribing technologies are sociocultural discourses that attempt to coerce the reader into accepting the reality constructed in the text.

The scientific inscription technologies of physical fitness exclude alternative accounts of the body. As I argued above, the body of fitness testing is produced under a disciplinary regime as an individual and a resource, and the reality recorded in the process is highly selective, looking only for signs that fit the paradigmatic (pouvoir) codes of the test. Information that does not fit the modern technological perspective of the codes is not recorded. Most important, information that could undermine the codes is left out. Indeed nothing of the body's puissance, its erotic reality, and the power of the BwO to deterritorialize its territorialization is recorded in the technologies of fitness confession. The coding of data is like the recording of a (digital) record that records only what the record company wants.

Take, for example, the fat that is recorded by the standard skinfold measurements of a fitness test. The test measures for adiposity in order to determine how functional the body–fat ratio is in accordance with population norms – determined by cadaver studies – as an epidemiology-based predictor of potential morbidity. The test does not record that the fatty 'love handles' (skinfold measurement at the iliac crest) could be much cherished by the participant-reader's lover as a site of erotic play and that just the night before they were intensely engaged in such play, dramatically deepening an erotic connection. The love handle may have been for one glorious moment a site for the deconstruction of individual difference and transgression of territorializing norms of human sexual behaviour. Nor does the test record the possibility that the participant-reader may fondly appreciate the fatty 'love handles' not only as a sign of increasing age, but as the embodiment of his or her acceptance of, or perhaps even erotic appreciation for, the feeling of growing older. This is not an insignificant point; for the test does not record anything that could challenge its resourceful paradigm of the body. It hides any questions of its disciplinary, individualizing, territorializing, resourcing paradigm. There is nothing in the structure of the test or in any part of its textual production that says: this is but one narrative of the body among many possible narratives, many of which you could write yourself, and some of which might completely undermine the presuppositions and priorities of this test.

Centring on the individual, supported by its circles, interactive texts such as fitness testing compel readers to confess themselves according to the cosmology of the modern self. The only language that the participant will hear is the language of modern sovereign self-hood. Imagine going to a physical fitness test and being asked about your eating and exercise habits, being prodded with fat calipers, being weighed on a scale, and doing sundry required exercises that will produce information on your body. Imagine saying to the appraiser/confessor: 'Don't ask me or "my body" to account; ask *our* BwO, the one that you and I are, the infinitely interdependent body of which we are reflections.' For all but the most brave, or mad, such a scenario is impossible. Called to account for 'oneself' in the language of the modern subject, surrounded by layers of technological texts and the exclusions of others, 'one' is likely to plug into the discourse, to confess what 'one' eats and how 'one' exercises, and to offer 'one's' fat, weight, and body movements to be measured.

Bazerman points out that the scientific control of knowledge production includes or excludes discourse, thereby determining what constitutes legitimate discourse within a scientific community. Such exclusion forms the encircling border that includes some texts and places others in their shadow. This happens paradigmatically – only those that share a particular paradigm join in the particular scientific discourse. Shapin and Schaffer also discuss this, pointing out that Britain's Royal Society was restricted to like-minded people who were willing to agree on the parameters of the debate. Similarly, fitness testing is produced in an exclusionary fashion: the only discourses that contribute to the creation and maintenance of the CPAFLA are those that share the paradigm of the body that I described above.

Alternative paradigms exist only in the shadow texts of the first three circles of texts. This exclusion is manifest in the complete absence from the first three circles of texts of any of the critical literature or perspectives. In reviewing the references in the second edition of the published guide to the CPAFLA (CSEP 1996), I found no evidence of philosophical, ideological, and political critiques of physical fitness and the science of physical fitness. Modifications to the new edition of 1996 attempted to bring more behavioural psychological concerns to the format, thus expanding the knowledge base beyond exercise physiology. But none of the behavioural references in that version mentions the critical literature. The only scholarly discourse that forms part of its scholarly background, as evidenced by references and the acknowledgments of contributors, is exercise science, defined narrowly by the biophysical, behavioural, and epidemiological sciences, without a hint of the critical social theories that have been developing in the social sciences and humanities for the last fifty years. The relegation of these critiques to the fourth order of texts minimizes dissent and makes possible a scientific consensus on physical fitness that does not take into account the power that science exercises through the body.

The establishment of authorial voice is crucial to the fitness test's capacity for symbolic violence. Of course, one technique for creating a domineering voice is simply to silence completely the reader. Fitness tests do that, while compelling the reader to believe that he or she has contributed to the text through his or her own bodily confessions. The truth that appears in the test is the truth of the participant, 'told' by him or her. In actuality, however, authorship is entirely by the CPAFLA: it disciplined the body to appear on the test's own terms, coded the body according to its own paradigm. As puissance, the BwO of the participant-reader has been entirely negated, symbolically erased from the text. The CPAFLA produces a text of pure pouvoir. This is the 'truth' that the participant-reader is asked to accept. The supreme authorial power, indeed magic, lies in hiding it all, leading the participant to believe that he or she has just seen the truth of his or her body.

It is very difficult to refute the 'truth' of a fitness appraisal. Participants are not privy to the calculations and the academic, institutional, and disciplinary cultures on which they are founded, which deal with the body paradigmatically as physical capital. The calculations are done by a computer, which effectively 'black boxes' the technical and socio-cultural complexities that lie behind them. Latour and Woolgar explain black-boxing as a technique that hides complexities so thoroughly that the reader cannot possibly appreciate the complexities and express doubt: 'The word *black box* is used by cyberneticians whenever a piece of machinery or a set of commands is too complex. In its place they draw a little black box about which they need to know nothing but its input and output' (Latour 1987, 2–3). Measurements are input to the black box of the computer and output on a simple scale of risk and benefit. The only thing that the participant (and the appraiser, for that matter) need be concerned about is input and output; the calculations and the entire field of science on which they are based, and the political and cultural priorities that developed that science, are unimportant. 'That is, no matter how controversial their history, how complex their inner workings, how large the commercial, [institutional] or academic networks that hold them in place, only their input and output count' (3).

That black box fully translates the participant's puissance (albeit poorly rendered in the disciplinary techniques of its measurement) into pouvoir, its value as physical capital in the accounting of risk and benefit. And the participant does not see it happen. In fact, because a computer does it, it is regarded as a simple, mundane, and technical process, not worthy of questioning. The essence of human being as puissance is reworked as pouvoir in the form of physical capital values of fitness, and it is rhetorically passed off as mere mechanical calculation! The transfiguration of human essence as pouvoir slips past in the rhetoric of mere technicality. A brilliant manoeuvre, really.

The questionnaires in popular texts also 'black box' the complexities of their appraisals. Palm-top computer fitness log books are tiny black boxes into which lives are compressed, cryptically reconfigured in the modernist cosmology, coded in the values of accumulation and lack, and 'outputted' to be read and further developed as resources. Credentiallizing in popular texts is seldom more extensive than the claim that they were designed by 'experts.' The ritual of truth here is very simple: the reader answers questions about himself or herself, and the answers tell a 'truth' about him or her. These popular forms, because they lack the controlling atmosphere of the fitness test, which is really the experimental laboratory transplanted, are not as thorough in their rhetoric and manipulative strategies. But, like the fitness test, so popular fitness questionnaires and log books compel the reader to confess according to the paradigms of the questionnaires, accounting for his or her physical accumulation of capital. Where the questionnaires focus on body shape, as in the vast majority in popular manuals and magazines, the meaning of the codes lies not so much in the physiological parameters of fitness as in the ways in which they account for the degree to which the reader's body has conformed to the iconographies of slimness, leanness, and muscularity, as constructed variously in norms of gender and race differences. As many other writers have documented, these normative cults of the fit body are so widespread and popular that they fulfil their own need for rhetorical power – that is, their omnipresence in itself makes them convincing. Just as the structuralist understanding of *vraisemblablisation* – the rhetorical power of common sense notions of reality – describes the power of machines to render truths about the body believable, so too norms of the fit-looking body make the codes of slenderness and muscularity appear to tell the truth of the body. Given the pervasiveness of the 'fit body' in popular culture, it would seem that it is the ageing, unfit body that is abnormal, unbelievable.

Confession is a technique of power that produces the body under the government of pouvoir as an individual, resourceful object that emits signs of itself, compelling it to account for itself in the abstract values of physical capital accumulation within the fundamental economy of lack that modern discourse inscribes. But accounting alone does not make modern subjectivity. Discipline is needed – and prescribed.

The central theme in my analysis of inscription has dealt with its productive power – the power of fitness testing, for instance, to bring the body to presence under pouvoir. This, I have argued, reproduces the culture of pouvoir, which is operative in the research laboratories of exercise science, which in turn reproduce the domineering cosmology of the modern subject. Brought to account in the logic of lack, the reader of these texts learns of the need for salvation from his or her own abjection. In the health-oriented texts, this is salvation from the risks of decay, death, and old age, the failing sovereignty of the non-self. In the appearance-oriented texts (such as fitness and fashion magazines), it is salvation from the abjection of not being 'beautiful,' young, self-confident, and self-possessed. The iconographic beauty of fit bodies is the beauty of perfection in the face of abjection: these compose an iconography that saves the sovereignty-seeking self from subordination to ageing, decay, and death.

Prescription

Writing Desire

Readers of physical fitness texts need to be saved from the void that the very idea of accounting presupposes. They need to develop their resources. 'Arbeit macht Frei.' As the Vivonic website points out: 'A recent study conducted by the Centers for Disease Control said that 80 million people start fitness programs each year and 95% fail because they lacked a plan, clear goals and a way to track their progress' (www.vivonic.com/video). The interactive texts offer a number of disciplinary techniques to get and keep the soteriological work project going. Through prescription, pouvoir achieves an ever-greater 'resolution' of its power (Foucault 1980a, 151–2): by inscribing a precise narrative for the production of future desire in individual bodies – for example, a particular workout program designed by a fitness appraiser for a specific individual. Pouvoir achieves greater resolution by prescribing techniques for 'lifestyles' dedicated to the development of physical capital in individual lives. There is an interesting cultural replay here. A broad cultural discourse of the body (pouvoir) that is generally circulating in modernity is reproduced in a highly controlled fashion in the research laboratory of exercise science, is reproduced again in the various inscribing technologies, and is then replayed (back) in the 'lifestyle' prescriptions that lay down strategies for living technologically, thus giving the general discourse of pouvoir greater 'resolution' in the wider culture.

Of course, daily life defies the sort of control possible in the laboratory. The research laboratory and fitness tests have scientists or appraisers, procedures and equipment, inscription devices and concrete texts, all of which control and record the movement of the body so that it is produced as resourcefully and accountably as possible. Power there is still operative externally. The body is marshalled as an object by an external subject (exercise scientist/appraiser). The trick of fitness counselling, indeed of a technological physical education, is to extend the control that marshals the body as a capital resource in the technologies of inscription into the day-to-day existence of individual, ostensibly self-determining, human subjects, over whom there is little if any external control in terms of resourceful fitness. It does that by writing a salvation narrative of the new life, which it calls a 'fit lifestyle' or 'healthy active living.' In the examination/confession, the power of pouvoir is momentary – the body is free to do as it wishes once it has performed its tasks, be they a set of push-ups or a guilty glance in the mirror. A technological physical education attempts to 'tight-couple' (Rouse 1987, 230) that *moment* of pouvoir by extending it beyond the limited spatio-temporal confines of a fitness appraisal in the form of an 'active day-to-day lifestyle.'

In 'Science and Reflection,' Heidegger (1953) speaks of a way of life that is geared not to dwelling on and beholding the essence of being – a way of dwelling that I have implied emerges in the alteritous practice of compassionate emptiness. He calls this other way of life the *bios praktikos*, 'the way of life that is dedicated to action and productivity' (165). The essence of 'lifestyle' for the technology of physical fitness is to produce human being by actions that focus on and increase its productivity as physical capital. Exercise and lifestyle prescription translates into action the abstract values of physical capital that are inscribed in the various assessing practices, such as fitness testing. It prescribes a way of life that compels the body to move as an individual functional object that can increase its value – a practical, functional, productive way of life, the bios praktikos. Counselling in fitness tests, by personal trainers, as well as popular manuals and exercise and dietary log books, produce texts that are scripts for the embodiment of the bios praktikos. This process encourages readers to read their bodies as practical texts and projects and to discipline them accordingly.

This is not just a matter of representation. Here is an appeal not just to *interpret* the body textually, as though there were many other equally important, valuable, or authentic interpretations. It is a matter of embarking on a textual production of the body such that it comes to be a *living* narrative of physical capital accumulation. This is the embodiment of scientific texts. Scripts are written for the body to become a simulacrum (Massumi 1997) of the modern subject. It is a textual strategy for the production of biopower.

This prescriptive writing of a 'lifestyle' is a textual attempt to 'make people up' by charting a disciplinary course for desire. The main technique involved here is panopticism (Foucault 1979, 195–230). Panopticism is a disciplinary technology that attempts to determine the essence of the body in the fundamental dynamics of puissance and pouvoir, scripting and monitoring how the body moves, how desire should be. I first outline Foucault's analysis of modern power as panoptic. I then describe some of the panoptics of the technology of physical fitness.

Through much of his work, Foucault has argued that modern coercive power is diffuse. No longer dependent on the concentrated great spectacles of power – such as public executions – modern power is exercised everywhere. The population co-operates extensively in the exercise of this power. In *Discipline and Punish*, Foucault (1979) analyses power as discipline that operates on individuals' bodies by making them docile, training them and overseeing them in a system that he calls 'panoptics.' The architectural archetype for this power was Jeremy Bentham's panopticon, which was a design for a prison that gave prisoners the impression that they could always be observed but that left them unable to detect when they were being observed. The disciplinary logic here was that they had to behave as if they were being watched all the time, even if they were not. The prisoners observed themselves on behalf of the prison. There was little need for jailers, since the prisoners themselves performed that function.

The panoptic form is not just architectural. It has become a social structure that has architectural manifestations, such as the prison, but which extends to many parts of life; it is a concept of control by surveillance in everyday life. It is a concept about surveillance by viewing, seeing, being aware of the constant possibility of being seen, and therefore disciplining oneself according to such seeing. It is a very cost-effective system that needs little in the way of a police force. Foucault (1980a) says: 'There is no need for arms, physical violence, material constraints. Just a gaze. An inspecting gaze, a gaze which each individual under its weight will end by interiorising to the point that he is his own overseer, each individual thus exercising this surveillance over, and against himself' (155).

The omnipresence of the fit body in visual culture has a panoptic effect, constantly reinforcing the image of slenderness, and so people watch over themselves for any deviations from slenderness. Foucault (1979) writes: 'He who is subjected to a field of visibility, and who knows it, assumes responsibility for the constraints of power; he makes them play spontaneously upon himself; he inscribes in himself the power relation in which he simultaneously plays both roles; he becomes the principle of his own subjection. By this very fact, the external power may throw off its physical weight; it tends to the noncorporal; and, the more it approaches this limit, the more constant, profound and permanent are its effects: it is a perpetual victory that avoids any physical confrontation and which is always decided in advance' (202–3). When power is effectively internalized, there is no confrontation with an other who is forcing one to do his or her bidding. Revolt becomes difficult because the oppressor cannot be seen. For this reason, panoptics brings a very low political cost to the 'regime.'

Mark Taylor (1990, 31ff) observes that the logic or reason of the panopticon is that of a deadline. In the spatial configurations of prisons, these deadlines are the physical boundaries that prisoners cross only at the risk of being shot. Temporally, deadlines are time limits, such as the time by which a debt must be paid or a work assignment must be submitted. Crossing a deadline can have serious consequences. Those who are aware of their deadlines and fearful of the consequences of not 'making' them organize their lives, their desires, their work in such a way that they do not cross the deadline. Like the panoptic jailer, the deadline operates in its own absence. 'The deadline is a THRESHOLD – an irreducible threshold that is never present as such. To cross the threshold is to run the risk of being shot – shot dead' (Taylor 1990, 31). Deadlines lurk in the presence of their absence as the threshold that must be avoided.

Prescriptive narratives, such as those written in fitness testing and exercise regimes, work with the logic of deadlines, thresholds that desire should not cross. Interactive texts write about thresholds that institute panoptic logic for desire. A number of thresholds are instituted. The most deadly is the threat of early death that might come from failing to produce enough physical capital to waylay the inevitable. Not as deadly, but certainly a threshold that one is encouraged not to cross, is the onset of disease, which results from poor accumulation of physical capital. Both death and disease are made present by their absence, thus threatening the participant. These deadlines are called 'health risks.' 'Health risks' become the absent panoptic jailer that keeps desire in check. Exposing oneself to health risk is the road not to be taken. The road to be taken is one of accumulating physical capital by increasing exercise, to improve cardiovascular function, and by perfecting body composition. With the absent deadline of health risk looming, one is given a text that prescribes a discipline for the production of desire: by diet, exercise, and ongoing panoptic monitoring.

The health risk deadline perpetually threatens that its absence will become presence if desire does not continue to unfold according to the prescription. For instance, when the appraisal of a fitness test tells a participant that there is no health risk for a particular component – for example, body composition – it adds: 'You are in no health risk with this score. It is important that your body composition not be allowed to shift toward being overfat as you age. A program of exercise and proper diet should be maintained.'[9] Foucault (1979) says: 'For the disciplined man, as for the true believer, no detail is unimportant, but not so much for the meaning that it conceals within it as for the hold it provides for the power that wishes to seize it' (140). Moreover, 'there is not a single moment of life from which one cannot extract forces, providing one knows how to differentiate it [sic] and combine it with others' (160).

Planning texts help readers rationally discipline their futures. The FITT principle organizes the frequency, intensity, type, and time of an exercise regime. Foucault's analysis of disciplinary time can be applied here. The first task is to establish a timetable: 'Time measured and paid must also be a time without impurities or defects; a time of good quality, throughout which the body is constantly applied to its exercise. Precision and application are, with regularity, the fundamental virtues of disciplinary time' (Foucault 1979, 149–51). The body's time is segmented into larger temporal configurations for the maximizing use of time over time, as it were: the exercise planners inscribe this as the 'time frame' – the number of weeks or months allotted to fulfilling fitness goals. The point here is to extract the body's resources over the long term, which, because the training effect is cumulative, is necessary to accumulate any meaningful physical capital.

Intensity, type, and time of the exercise constitute what Foucault calls the 'temporal elaboration of the act.' Within the exercise regimen, the body's time must not be permitted to break out on its own, to be inefficient. The ITT of the FITT principle ensures development of maximal resources. The ITT is calculated to ensure that just the right amount of work is performed. Intensity here is a rational matter. It is not prescribed as a deterritorializing plateau, as Deleuze and Guattari (1987) speak of the liberating power of (erotic) intensities (149–66) (see discussion in chapter 2, above). The intensity must not be so great that it might undermine the (territorializing) capital project – for instance, people running very fast for four minutes may experience profound erotic, indeed deterritorializing intensity; but if that activity completely tires them so that they cannot run longer and achieve the training effect, their energy, their puissance, their time has been 'wasted.' The ITT maximizes the body's resourcefulness. Foucault (1979) says that this sort of discipline 'poses the principle of a theoretical ever-growing use of time: exhaustion rather than use; it is a question of extracting, from time, ever more available moments and, from each moment, ever more useful forces. This means that one must seek to intensify the use of the slightest moment, as if time, in its very fragmentation, were inexhaustible or as if, at least by an ever more detailed internal arrangement, one could tend towards an ideal point at which one maintained maximum speed and maximum efficiency' (154). Maximum efficiency in resource management is the ideal embodiment of the modern subject of the technology of physical fitness.

Salvation and Consumption

The intertextual ensemble reveals the body, brings it to presence as a resource. The goal of this resourcing of the body is to make it ever more productive and efficiently functional, so that it is more fully useful. Developing the use-value of puissance as pouvoir is the point of this technology. The wonder, the ecstasy, the intrinsic value of puissance is entirely irrelevant. There is but one imperative: to increase the physical capital value of the individual body by developing physical fitness. The ensemble prescribes the instrumental rationale for maximizing the body's capital potential. Accumulated physical capital purchases salvation in various forms. I briefly describe the forms of salvation that development of physical capital is supposed to purchase. I seek not so much to embellish themes developed well by others as to illustrate how exercise technology and exercise science serve larger socio-cultural discourses that use the body as a resource. Remember that the genius of this technology is its ability to capture the wild, spontaneous, erotic power of the BwO, by territorializing it in the confessional and disciplinary process.

The scientific capital resourcing of puissance is instrumental to many of the socio-cultural projects that the critical literature of physical fitness has addressed. Foremost among these, perhaps, is individualism, which I have described as egocentrism. I have shown above that the capital resource development of the technology of physical fitness deals exclusively with the production of the body as an individual capital resource. For instance, the individualism of workplace fitness programs, which often revolve around fitness testing as a 'motivational tool,' encourages employees to develop their bodies as more productive capital resources, exhibiting increased productivity, lower absenteeism, and more placid dispositions (Shephard 1986). The transfer of 'responsibility' for health from the state to the individual saves the state from having to care for its citizens (Harvey 1983; 1988; Harvey, Beamish, and Defrance 1993; Ingham 1985; H. Stein 1982). 'Saving' the state money has been a major impetus for the 'lifestyle' improvement strategies of health promotion. Many of those campaigns press 'individuals' to take responsibility for their health. My analysis above shows that, in the technology of physical fitness, individuals, doing so means developing their bodies as personal physical capital.

The technology of physical fitness reproduces the ideology of bourgeois individualism that pervades modern consumer culture (Glassner 1989; H. Stein 1982). Salvation is best understood here in terms of the perils of lack that it seeks to avoid. The following is a summary of the various discourses of the body that others have studied, applied to my analysis of modern soteriology. Accumulating physical capital in the slender, taut body saves one from the judgment by peers of being lazy, unproductive, undisciplined, self-indulgent, emotionally unstable, and so on (Bordo 1990; Robert Crawford 1984; Trish Crawford 1995; Featherstone 1991). Men can save themselves from the ignominy of femininity by building their masculine physical capital in large muscles (Bordo 1999; Connell 1990; Pronger 1992; Whitson 1994). By becoming strong, women can save themselves from the sexist imperative that they remain weak (Cole 1993; Lloyd 1996; MacNeill 1994; Markula 1995; Martin 1989; Moore 1997), or conversely they can embody a patriarchal culture's distaste for a woman's body by exercising to disappear – the twisted logic of anorexia nervosa described by Bordo (1993, 139–64). Engaging in the consumer cultures of physical fitness, fantasizing about, shopping for, and purchasing fitness products and services, saves one from the dissatisfaction of not consuming. Salvation here is the meaning to be found in the act of consumption itself: 'I consume, therefore I am.' One can save oneself from the dissatisfaction with self fostered by consumer culture, particularly through advertising images, by working on one's body (Featherstone 1991; Falk 1994). One can earn salvation from loneliness and sexual inadequacy by building the physical capital of the sexy, 'fit' body (Lelwica 1999). Physical capital development promises to save one from an early death, from sickness, and from the ravages of old age. The imperative to be young and to buy youth through fitness is omnipresent. Indeed, looking one's age is a sign of a failure to accumulate youthful physical capital. The technology of physical fitness marshals the body as a capital resource for the purchase of these soteriological ends.

I am not arguing here that physical fitness cannot deliver many of the promises listed above. It can. In some cases it does. The problem, I suggest, is that this form of salvation transforms desire as a positive life-force, the essence of the non-limitive BwO, and reterritorializes it in the logic of lack. The impetus to move (i.e., the being of desire) comes not from the infinity of what the body is (One Bright Pearl, infinite reflection), but from the finitude of what it is not (sovereign subject). The soteriological quest here is to embody fantasy, to come to presence as what one is not: beautiful, productive, masculine, feminine, forever young, healthy, fully alive. In short, it promises to save one from reality. It promises to purchase the fantasies of being what one is not and of not becoming what one inevitably will become.

This fantasy of purchasing what one lacks is the heart of the desire to accumulate physical or any other kind of capital. This fantasy is the very engine of consumer capitalism: dissatisfaction with what is present and an unrequitable longing for what is absent. The basis of consumer desire is lack: the impoverished presence of desiring absence. Puissance, I have argued, is its opposite: it is the erotic, fecund intensity of presence, which exists in the absence of lack, a paradoxical intensity that is ultimately the reality of emptiness. The basis of personal capital accumulation, in contrast, is unrequitable desire. For when desire moves in the empty, smooth space of the BwO, the open Body of Reality, it has no need to move in the mode of accumulation. Movement that does not need to accumulate anything is free; movement that needs to accumulate is bound to the project. The movements prescribed in the technology of physical fitness are bound by the logic of accumulation, not free. The economics of consumer capitalism requires the ironic desire to lack. The imperative to physical capital accumulation, which is the essence of movement in exercise science, reproduces the structure of desire (as unrequitable lack) in consumer capitalism. Desire, in the science of physical fitness, is always unrequitable because it is always produced in the fear of its panoptic deadlines – the abject risk of failed sovereignty. This lackful desire is consummated, ironically enough, only past the threshold of death itself. In death, I suspect, there are no health risks, at least not as conceived by the science of physical fitness.

The enticement to accumulate physical capital for the purchase of bodily fantasy territorializes the puissant body with the pouvoir of lack. The capitalist imperative is always to be richer, no matter how rich or poor you are. The magnet of capital accumulation through physical fitness is the power of lack, of absence, of the nihilistic purchase of life.

I am not saying that there is anything wrong with living a long time, free of disease, and irresistibly attractive. What is wrong is desire brought to presence, territorialized by pouvoir, negating puissance, by constructing desire as lack. This, I believe, adds to Heidegger's warning about the danger of modern technology – that it does not attend to beings coming to presence from themselves and instead marshals them as mere resources for other uses (Gestell). In the logic of individual capital accumulation, the body/desire comes to presence by the negation of its infinity. Salvation through accumulation of physical (fitness) capital is a technology that brings desire to presence by the draw of its own negation. The nasty irony of finding salvation in capital accumulation is that one is saved by the loss of the fulness of the BwO, by the seduction of lack. The 'healing power,' the source of salvation in this strange narrative, turns out to be nihilism, the negation of the fulness of presence in desire. The science and technology of physical fitness prescribe this nihilism under the code words 'healthy lifestyle,' which, from Heidegger's perspective, can be understood as the *bios praktikos*.

The word 'lifestyle' was originally used by Alfred Adler to denote structures of the personality that govern reactions and behaviour. Adler saw this governing structure as being established in the first four or five years of an individual's life. For exercise science, lifestyle is also a governing structure, but not one that is patterned on early childhood development, a kind of predestination that comes from childhood. The 'healthy lifestyle' of exercise science is a panoptic government of life, a relentless project of confession (monitoring fitness) and resolution to subjection (writing and following prescriptions for exercise and controlling desire). Unlike Adler's predestination, exercise science produces lifestyle in an ongoing project of discipline, panopticism, and denial that extends that paradigm of the body from the rarefied confines of the research laboratory into every moment of everyday life. A healthy lifestyle is a 'boundary project' (Haraway 1985) that channels desire (Deleuze and Guattari 1987, 33) in the production of pouvoir. For a healthy lifestyle, desire follows guidelines for eating, sleeping, exercising, drinking, lovemaking, working ... There is no part of life, no detail too small (Foucault 1979, 140), that it cannot be bounded by the disciplinary gaze of lifestyle management.

The term 'healthy lifestyle' is pregnant with morality. H. Stein (1982) points out: 'The inflection and doggedness with which "health" is promoted and disease prevented gives the whole show away. Substitute perdition for disease, and salvation for health (or "wellness") and one lays bare the old morality play, here replayed in the idiom of medicine. We are admonished and instructed to restore our bodies and spirits to health through vigorous exercise (running and jogging, for instance), through various abstinences, meditation, and the like. If we adhere to this self-discipline, we will purge our bodies and minds of those poisons that make us ill. We will thereby become clean, healthy – saved' (169).

'Lifestyle' is an individual 'consumer choice' with powerful moral implications. One 'chooses' to be healthy or unhealthy, moral or immoral, normal or deviant. The imperative is to choose the right lifestyle, channel desire to avoid the abyss of deviance: 'The notion of deviancy is extended from the sick person to the potentially sick person, from manifest illness to what is considered unhealthy behaviour. We all become deviants in our everyday lives – when we light up a cigarette, when we consume eggs at breakfast, and when we are unable to express fully our emotions. Persons who act in such a way as to predispose themselves to sickness are now considered actually to be sick. Like the sick role, the potential-sick role mandates a moral duty: to correct unhealthy habits. Conversely, it condemns illness as an individual moral failing' (Robert Crawford 1980, 380). The individualist focus of lifestyle withdraws the body from the puissance of the essential connectedness of the prepersonal, of finding salvation in the profoundly connected puissance of desire, and moves it into the pouvoir of the controlled, self-disciplined territory of bourgeois individual accumulation of physical capital. Producing this individuality is constructed as a moral duty.

The clarion call of the 'healthy lifestyle' is to pursue a way of life that is devoted to the practicalities of capital accumulation – a *bios praktikos*.[10] I conclude this chapter commenting on the problems of the bios praktikos as a way of life. In regard to the body, the bios praktikos is a simulacrum of the body, a partial concretization of its potential, that deals with it exclusively as a practical matter of developing physical capital resources for the sovereign project. This way completely obscures the dynamics of puissance and pouvoir, passing off the territorializing power of pouvoir as nothing more than a natural account of the body. The *bios praktikos* hides the operations of power both in science and in the modern technological making of day-to-day life. In the specific case of fitness testing, I have shown above that it accomplishes this hiding through acts of considerable symbolic violence.

The transformative power of scientific technology is its ability to make worlds, according to the paradigms of science (Rouse 1987, 211). The CPAFLA, for instance, was designed to transform human life, to produce a *made* world from an epidemiological point of view – one of the primary motivations of health promotion and, since 1974, a policy of the Canadian government, as of many other 'developed countries.' But this transformative power is also the making of individual, individualized worlds that are subject to authoritative, resourceful discourses on the body, discourses of which the participants are not made aware and to which they are not invited to contribute, except by their docile embodiment of them – participants undergoing fitness testing have no say in the writing of the narrative of their desire. They provide a certain kind of data (and in highly restricted forms) that is then organized according to external discourse. But the rhetorical hope, of course, is that these discourses will become internalized so that participants understand themselves along the narrative lines imposed and come to embody the narrative, thus internalizing the discourse. Plugged into the discourse, new worlds emerge.

Where exercise science is the dominant episteme of physical education, reflections on the body's puissance are done considerable violence. The bios praktikos becomes common sense, or what Bourdieu has called a 'habitus,' a habitual 'system of schemes of perception, thought, appreciation and action' (Bourdieu and Passeron 1990, 35) about the body's being. This habitus, of course, circulates throughout modern capitalist culture, especially in the upper and middle classes, and above all for men. The bios praktikos of physical education reproduces a habitus that is already in circulation. Thoughtful reflection on the body, critical awareness of the way in which technology marshals it, gives way to the common sense of the bios praktikos.

Failure to reflect on the dynamics of puissance and pouvoir, to appreciate the territorialization of puissance by pouvoir, amounts to a failure to see the body's power as puissance, to appreciate its potential for freedom, its non-individualist constitution in the infinitely interdependent reflective body, the non-limitive BwO. This failure amounts to living in the shadow of the essence of technology, rather than in the light of the essence of the body as moving being: free, infinite. By continuing to live in such a shadow, without reflecting on the light that is withheld by it, we fail to fulfil our most fundamental responsibilities as beings who have the capacity to care for the way in which we and our fellow beings come to presence in our puissant essence. It is a way of life for the pure resourcing of the body. And it plays to the dynamics of resource and waste product as well. Physical education of the bios praktikos attends only to the body's resourcefulness, casting off its puissant freedom. In fact, where people most fully pursue the bios praktikos, where pouvoir is totally active, puissance becomes entirely physical capital, subjected completely to the government of pouvoir.

Conclusion

The technologies of description, inscription, and prescription mortify the body, reproducing long-standing Christian traditions. Quoting Foucault, Zygmunt Bauman (1998) says: 'All those Christian techniques of examination, confession, guidance, obedience, have an aim: to get individuals to work at their own "mortification" in this world. Mortification is not death, of course, but is a renunciation of this world and oneself; a kind of everyday death. A death which is supposed to provide life in another world' (59). Slightly rewritten, this point is prescient for my deconstruction of the technology of physical fitness. The modern techniques of description, inscription, and prescription have an aim: to get individuals to work at their own 'mortification' of being in this world. Mortification is not death, of course, but is a renunciation of the essential freedom and infinity of puissance, a kind of everyday death, for the sake of sovereignty. Because such sovereignty is actually full subjection, it is fascist.

In chapter 2, I wrote: 'By fascism I mean the desire to order, organize, control, repress, direct, impose limits, to interrupt the free flow of desire so as to subordinate it to pouvoir. Fascism crystallizes the popular desire to be led, to be the subject of power. So this fascism is a *will* within us to desire, albeit often unwittingly, a life of domination.' This life of domination is the sovereign life written in the texts of the technology of physical fitness. Where might it lead?

Postscript: The Other Side

For the issue depends on Freedom: and it is in the power of freedom to pass beyond any and every specified limit.

Immanuel Kant, *Critique of Pure Reason*

The technology of physical fitness writes a relatively coherent script for the body, suggesting limited and productive directions for desire. I have argued above that it is a script not for freedom, but for subjection to the modernist quest for sovereignty, for salvation in a life described as essentially lacking. The intertextual ensemble writes codes for the resourcing of puissance by pouvoir. These texts are not alone in their reproduction of the trajectory of the modern human subject. They make sense and are applicable because they represent a particular manifestation of a larger project that is at work in many spheres of modern life. They attempt to bring ever-greater resolution to the subjection of life to the domineering project of resource management and exploitation. While it is possible for people to engage in the physicality of exercise and experience realities that move beyond the reproduction of the modern subject, the intertextual ensemble described above does not foster such a beyond; the ensemble renders it second in the parergonality of the technology. As I mentioned above in the Preface, that was my personal experience of exercise – I became physically active in order to accumulate physical capital and inadvertently discovered the infinite potential of the body. But everywhere I looked in the intertextual ensemble for help and understanding of the depth and infinity to which I had been awakened, I found only more subjection.

In this Postscript, I consider first where the technology directs or orients its readers and practioners, and, drawing on the theory of the body from chapter 2, I ask whether this approach to the body offers any potential for alterity so that we may move beyond nihilism (the second subject of this Postscript) and towards transcendence (the third subject).

I present here only a preliminary sketch of principles for alterity. Suggesting concrete strategies and analysing existing practices (such as the contemplative martial arts, yoga, tantra, and somatics) constitute a major undertaking that I leave to another volume. My consideration here needs to be a reflective practice in which we consider the nature of alterity within the modern technological approach to the body. My focus above has been to deconstruct the *texts* of the technology of physical fitness, and I have left open the empirical question of the extent to which they have been successful in actually territorializing the lived experience of our Body without Organs (BwO). A broad empirical account of the actualization of the technologization of the BwO is beyond the scope of this book and is also best left to another volume. But I think that we can use the analytical tools that I have been developing throughout this book to reflect on our own embodiments and to discern the interplay of puissance and pouvoir and thereby get a sense of at least the potential for alterity there.

Reflecting on our situation is very difficult for a number of reasons. It is emotionally difficult work because it means looking into our BwO and reflecting deeply on the state of our desires, for the ways in which they embody humanism, egocentrism, youth-centrism, and phallocentrism, for instance. It means looking into our collective soul, as it were, and being prepared to confront something terrible. Taylor (1987) asks: 'Is it possible to fathom the darkness exposed in the midst of the high noon of modernity?' (41). The dynamic interrelations of pouvoir and puissance mean that nothing is clear-cut. As I wrote in chapter 2, pouvoir resources puissance in order to become puissant. The result is that even where territorialization is thorough, there is the essential freedom of becoming. Our task, therefore, is to discern what is happening in this interrelationship of puissance and pouvoir. As Glass observes of enlightened practice, it means becoming sensitive to the whole (the wave of light/puissance) in the particular (the particle of light/pouvoir).

It may be that the current North American mania for exercise and diet may actually end up not serving its 'proper' purpose in making docile and disciplined human subjects. Just as in early modern Christianity the popularity of the macabre led some religious to find pleasure there, so too the popularity of 'no pain, no gain,' may represent a departure 'from the moral and religious lesson [to] a gradual sliding into sadistic pleasure' (Delumeau 1990, 112–13). What begins as a reterritorializing strategy can turn out to be deterritorializing. Is this not perhaps the case in the 'extreme' training that is part of the cult of the marathon, the triathlon, the iron man competition, and other 'extreme' sports? Is there in painful pleasure, in the intensity of hard training, a path out of body fascism by the very technology of its institution (Dillard 1999, 51)?

My emphasis on the historical organization of desire in modernity could be (mis)read as nostalgic – if only we could return to a more pristine, 'natural' way that antedates the ravages of modernity. This is not possible. There is nowhere else to go. Modernity is our context. Moreover, I do not think that there was ever a better time to live and reflect, and things are not going to get any better in the future. Annie Dillard (1999) puts it well: 'There were no formerly heroic times, and there was no formerly pure generation. There is no one here but us chickens, and so it has always been: a people busy and powerful, knowledgeable, ambivalent, important, fearful, and self-aware; a people who scheme, promote, deceive, and conquer; who pray for their loved ones, and long to flee misery and escape death. It is a weakening and discolouring idea, that rustic people knew God personally once upon a time – or even knew selflessness or courage or literature – but that it is too late for us. In fact, the absolute is available to everyone in every age. There never was a more holy age than ours, and never less (88).

It is important that this reflection on alterity within technology not be grounded (Nancy 1993) in either nostalgia or false optimism. From an ecological point of view, our BwO is suffering, and momentous changes are occurring. Human development over the last century has transformed our 'environment,' other species, and the overall ecosystem. Depending on whom you listen to, these effects range from debilitating but recoverable to a complete disaster, bringing life on the planet to the edge of collapse. Many forms of life have already disappeared as a direct result of modern human development. The litany of problems is familiar: acid rain destroying forest and lake habitats;

global supplies of fresh water diminishing rapidly; rain forests disappearing; thousands of species vanishing; biodiversity diminishing;
global warming bringing devastating wild weather conditions; and a
veritable time bomb of nuclear waste waiting to be unleashed, which
some of it already has been in Russia.

While I am by no means an expert on the complicated business of
predicting the various outcomes of all these ecological problems both
separately and as they will no doubt affect one another in chaotic
fashion, there seems to be no indication that the destruction is going
to stop. For instance, the number of species on Canada's endangered
list has doubled since 1988; and emissions of carbon dioxide (which
spur global warming) have risen in North America by 14 per cent
since 1990, and at the time of writing neither Canada nor the United
States is willing to fulfil its obligations under the Kyoto Protocol. In
May 2001, the U.S. Vice-President Dick Cheney announced that American demand for electricity in the next twenty years will increase by 43
per cent, and that the U.S. administration's policy is not to curtail
those 'demands': 'Conservation may be a sign of personal virtue but it
is not a sufficient basis for a sound, comprehensive energy policy'
(Cambell 2001). Instead, the Americans plan to fill their demand for
more energy by more aggressive exploitation of traditional fuels: oil,
natural gas, coal, and nuclear energy. Furthermore, their plans for
military domination, including in outer space, articulate an aggressive
attitude that is about more than purely military defence. Humanist
economic expansion is the name of the game.

And this is not just a Euro–American phenomenon. The so-called
developing world is trying to pull itself from poverty and play the
game that we in the 'developed world' are playing. There is little
indication that that will change. This scenario of ecological degradation and potential ultimate collapse is eschatalogical: it understands
our experience of life and the future in terms of endings, last things,
final possibilities. We live perhaps in an eschatalogical environment,
which is coming to its end and taking us with it.

In this well-known scenario of ecological destruction there are many
people who agree with its diagnosis and who still work with hope for
a solution to the problem, a strategy that will resist these changes. If
we can just come up with the right conceptual framework, if we can
just convince the right people, if we can just develop the right eco-
friendly technologies, if we can just make the right economic adjust-

ments, and so on, we can slow and eventually change the disastrous direction in which humanity and life on earth are otherwise inexorably heading. I see no justification for that kind of hope. While my reluctance to join the eco-optimist club comes from my reading the ecological 'facts' as being just so dire that that attitude strikes me as deluded; I also appreciate that predicting the future is very difficult and that there are so many contingencies that it really is impossible to know what is going to happen. The modern aggressive technological approach that is ruining the ecosphere is also reflected in the modern technological approach to the body.

I would therefore like to approach the problem in a different way. Rather than looking out to the environment and the future, I suggest looking in to the ways in which we are constructed now. This should be a reflective undertaking. The myth of Indra's Net is helpful to this task. Recalling that each jewel in the net reflects all the other jewels infinitely, we can reflect on how the technological approach to the body reflects the modern aggressive approach to life on the planet. The destructiveness that that approach takes to creation reflects the infinite wave of the universe, which is ultimately both creative and destructive, fraught with both presence and absence – a relationship that, as Heidegger has observed, is essential to movement and, as Dōgen has said, is the nature of impermanence, which Buddhist perspectives see as the ultimate nature of reality.

The optimism that supposes that we can fix the mess into which we have gotten ourselves, that we can cling to the past by taking control of the future, is the false optimism of modernity. As I argued in chapter 3, this modernity enshrines humanity as the architect both of its potential disastrous fate and of its potential salvation. Whereas Christian eschatology entrusted the fate of the world to a domineering, patriarchal God, its modern successor, atheistic technological humanism, supposes that humanity has the power that used to be the providence of God to save itself and the rest of the world. Modernity reworks the Christian soteriology that pictures the eschatological fate of the world as lying between the power of God and the freedom of humans to choose good over evil, eternal bliss over damnation. Modernity reworks that soteriology as lying with the power of technological humanity to choose the right course for the longevity of individuals, the species, and the environment. It depends on our making canny, rational choices. This is the familiar reasoning of the European

Enlightenment – that momentous philosophical, spiritual, and material shift that has us desire the very thing that is destroying us and seemingly everything that we touch. It is the phallic desire for control.

I have argued above that the modern desire for sovereignty is in fact a desire for subjection and that that desire is fascist. And the disciplinary techniques of physical fitness, which attempt to rein in the essential freedom of the movement of the body in the ironic quest for sovereignty through subordination, are the techniques of body fascism. The fully fascist body comes to presence where the body is entirely subjected to the power of pouvoir. The more purely physical education focuses on the resourcing *bios praktikos*, 'the way of life that is dedicated to action and productivity' (Heidegger 1953, 165: Bataille, 1986 #202, similarly), rather than on a way of life dedicated to reflection, the *bios theoreticos*, the more it tends to embody fascism, which today is the body subjected entirely to the resourceful embodiment of capitalist desire (Hocquenghem 1995, 260).

The ubiquitous representation of the fit body in consumer culture is the iconography of body fascism. When we read our own bodies and the bodies of others by reference to such iconography – i.e., beautiful or desirable for the way in which it conforms to the iconography, and ugly or undesirable for its deviations – we subject the body's limitless potential to its manifestation of fascist desire. As Deleuze (1992) observes: 'People in a society desire repression, both for others and "for themselves." There are always people who want to bug others and who have the opportunity, the "right" to do so' (1992). Consider the keen desire of the Canadian government to 'change the values of Canadians' and of the Canadian Society for Exercise Physiology (1996) to 'trigger changes and influence the personal health practices of clients [and to] in turn improve their coping skills and give them a greater sense of mastery and control over their lives' (1–3) – for their own good, of course. Consider also the well-intentioned prods of friends and lovers who suggest that one is putting on weight, proffering advice on diets and exercise.

Nihilism

Where does body fascism take us? Its parergonal product is nihilism, erasure of the limitless BwO, negation of the 'Body of Reality,' closure on the freedom of movement. The open, free space of movement is foreclosed by the centrisms of the modern subject that I described in chapter 3. Body fascism includes the particle and precludes the wave field of perception. It works most effectively when people live and think predominantly in particle reality rather than in wave reality. And it is at its most effective when the wave is beyond imagination, where life is devoted to the particle. The intertextual ensemble of the technology of physical fitness renders the wave second. Before moving to that secondness, and the alteritous potential that is there, I wish to reflect on the nihilism of body fascism.

The individualism of the technology of physical fitness is problematic, as Ingham has argued, because it does not adequately address the unequal distribution of opportunities for physical activity and, as Laberge has maintained, because it hegemonizes a middle-class habitus. But I would say that it is more profoundly problematic because it does not foster the deeper attunement to Being/becoming as a whole (the non-limitive BwO) and our consequent essential interconnectedness. As such it constitutes the body negatively, denying the truth of Being/becoming, fostering nihilism. Nihilism might be associated with the path of material human-made ecospherical destruction that we see advancing across the surface of the planet, rapidly changing life as we know it. But following a fundamental Buddhist insight on impermanence, I suggest that nihilism is instead the aggressive human refusal to live in the truth of movement, which is presence fraught with absence, creation with destruction, ultimate radical impermanence. Nihilism is the denial of impermanence and is expressed in the grasping human and phallic desire to take control over it. Nihilism harbours enmity towards impermanence rather than compassion. For compassion joins in the passion of impermanence, of movement, *Eriegnis*, rather than turning away. The destruction of the ecosphere is the product of our nihilism.

Nihilism is closure to that which is beyond sovereign humanism. Heidegger postulates that this closure results from the modernist tendency to reflect on reality not as it is *in-itself* but rather as it is perceived in human subjectivity. The in-itself, he says, disappears. It disappears both in the positive sciences and in modern technology, which call on the grounding of humanism to perceive and make reality according to human desire. The in-itself also disappears in what we might call the strong program of social constructionism, which sees all perception (and therefore reality production) as thoroughly dependent on human social constructions. Heidegger says that this annihilation of the in-itself serves the domineering, resourcing desires of modern humanity. It is inspired by the death of God and by the ascent of Man.

Nihilism, then, is produced in humanity's will to power. I have described this above as the project of sovereignty, whose emotional logic is fear of that which is beyond human, ego, and phallus – fear of difference. For this reason the most modern human is concerned primarily with himself or herself and with whatever furthers that self and produces its identity. This, of course, is precisely the call of physical fitness. Ostensibly, the less one hears that is beyond the self, the more comfortable one is, the less fearful one is. Taylor (1984) explains that nihilism is 'the nothingness of consciousness when consciousness becomes the foundation of everything. Man the murderer of God and drinker of the sea of creation wanders through the infinite nothingness of his own ego' (32). In 'Teaching a Stone to Talk,' Annie Dillard (1982) despairs of the modern Western ability to hear nature speak. This deafness to nature means that we hear only the shrieking of modern humanity. It precludes the power of reflection that would allow us to understand ourselves transpersonally, transpecially, transmorphically. It annihilates our ability to live fully in the free, unbounded spatiality of the non-limitive BwO, which Dōgen calls the Body of Reality, the One Bright Pearl of impermanence.

The philosophy of the limit seeks to undermine what Cornell (1992) calls the 'ideology of lesser expectations' (17). The ideology of lesser expectations is at work in configurations that limit the possibilities of life to a given system, such as the technology of physical fitness. But Cornell says that there is a 'more-than-this' dimension, something more than what is presented by particular configurations of possibility that circulate discursively. There is, for instance, 'more-than-this' in the gendered identity of being a woman or a man. I suggest that there is a 'more-than-this' to physical activities such as running that transcends the humanism, egocentrism, youth-centrism, and phallocentrism that I discussed in chapter 3. The ideology of lesser expectations is a fundamentally conservative/reactionary ideology that promotes accepting the thin gruel that modern consumer capitalist patriarchy markets as 'quality of life' and 'lifestyle choice,' for instance. By setting the bar very low, as it were, this ideology aids the resourcing of puissance by pouvoir. The pervasiveness in late modernity of people living finite lives, not really imagining the infinite as anything more personally significant to them than the abstract musings of mathematicians and physicists, attests to lesser expectations. The primacy of self and human shows the expectation of very little indeed.

The fact that the technology of physical fitness gives virtually no consideration beyond the finite concerns of egocentric and anthropocentric individuals is testimony to its lesser expectations. And its dominance in physical education expresses modern society's low expectations for educating the body. The most that one can expect from identifying with technology is desire as lack, body fascism. As a counter to this worldview, Cornell suggests the revelation of the 'more-than-this' in non-identity. This means developing the realization that there is more happening in the body than the representations of the technology of physical fitness would suggest. It *is* possible to *not* identify with modern sovereigntist technological paradigms of the body.

Transcendence

The technology of physical fitness has misrepresented the puissance of our BwO as a resource for the sovereign project. But it also goes further than simply *representing* the body: through the processes of description and inscription it attempts to *make* puissance a resource. But, as I argued above in my theory of the body, we are moving in the sphere of puissance, regardless of our technological take on it. The point is to attend to puissance and to let *it* play freely, to let the in-itself of puissance simply happen. This does not mean abandoning modernity and the technologies that appear to be indispensable for most humans now, but it involves living and seeing through the pouvoir of technology to realize puissance. What we need is the ability to become more than technological. We must foster the alterity that lurks in the secondness of technological parergonality.

I suggest that we need to move, to be embodied, in post-technological ways. As in post-colonialism (Ashcroft, Griffiths, and Tiffin 1995, 117), the 'post' of the post-technological is not a time that comes after the technological era, but a way of living within technology that is not limited by it. Post-technological approaches can offer openings for resistance to the technologization of the body from within the technological project. In this sense it is not utopian. It looks for opportunities for resistance and transcendence within overarching discourses that annihilate such possibilities. It is a matter of living within body fascism while being less of it. For embodiment, even under fascism, 'is not a curse, not an affliction, but the only opportunity we shall be given to learn the poetry of mortal dwelling' (Levin 1985, 68). And what is the poetry of *mortal* dwelling, if not the 'one bright pearl' of impermanence?

Part of seeing through our nihilism is working with it, not just escaping it. This stance entails engaging the melancholy of negative dialectics. 'The melancholy science is not one of defeat; to be melancholic is to experience deprivation as loss. This is itself a form of resistance in a world in which deprivation [desire as lack] is justified as necessary' (Cornell 1992, 30). Realizing deprivation, rather than avoiding it, one can move beyond it. As the contemplative Thomas Merton said: 'What we have to be is what we are' (as cited in Johnson 1998, 39). So just as the construction of desire as lack is a technique for our subjection to being incomplete subjects who engage in modern technologies of salvation, so too that lack, seen for what it is, offers us the opportunity to be open to difference and to move beyond domination. Recognizing the ways in which body fascism shapes desire begins the process of clearing away the obstacles to the sensual ease that can be the very nature of the smooth, free space of the deterritorializing BwO. In this context we can associate Glass's reading of emptiness – as a practice of compassionate openness to the alterity of the wave – with the body's learning sensual ease, moving in the free space of movement that is not tied to the desire for domination.

While Bataille's work on eroticism frequently conveys a violence that would seem to be at odds with the peaceful acceptance that Glass's work on emptiness connotes, there are aspects of it that illuminate secondness and the potential for transcendence. Bataille is interested in what systems leave out, what they expel, their 'excretions.' He proposes that what systems leave out gives them a blind spot; for what they omit is no longer part of their vision. But it is precisely by looking through the blind spot that transcendence of the system becomes possible. By apprehending that which body fascism leaves out, we can approach the body's alteritous possibilities. It is precisely that which the system of modern subject formation renders second – that capacity of sacred awareness that is not itself observed with the panoptic gaze – that makes possible transcendence of the nihilism of modernity. In *Inner Experience*, Bataille (1988) writes: 'When I solicit gently, in the very heart of anguish, a strange absurdity, an eye opens itself at the summit, in the middle of my skull. This eye which, to contemplate the sun, in its nudity, face to face, opens up to it in all its glory, does not arise from my reason: it is a cry that escapes me. For at that moment when the lightning stroke blinds me, I am the flash of a broken life, and this life – anguish and vertigo – opening itself up to an infinite void, is lacerated and spends itself all at once in this void, (as cited in Taylor 1987, 123).

The sacredness of infinity is the excrement of the modern subject. Certainly this is the excrement of the technology of physical fitness, which focuses entirely on the finite individual human subject. And in modernity, attending to this 'excrement' has precisely the status of playing with shit. But, ironically enough, by entering modernity's excrement, one can transcend its dominating power.

Bataille is also very interested in the body's holes, its gapiness. The body can excrete because it has openings. The body's orifices point to the fact that the body does not live with tidy distinctions of interior and exterior, distinctions that are critical for the modern, self-contained – i.e., sovereign – subject. The muscular, taught, technologically constructed body signifies sovereignty, impermeability, the enclosed body from which nothing escapes the panoptics of fitness. The fit body is proper, clean, neat, and tidy – it is a body that resists the transgressive capacity of the 'gaping body' to allow difference. The cult of the tight body is the cult of a body that does not give way to the other. Jiggly flesh is obscene, ugly because it gives flesh to the body's malleability, its lack of sovereignty when it is prodded or even when it moves. It suggests that the flesh has a life of its own, oblivious to the will of the sovereign subject. Just as the sovereign God that Michelangelo depicted on the ceiling of the Sistine Chapel is large, hard, and muscular – it is unimaginable that he would be fat, jiggly, loose, out of control – so too God's successor, the modern, sovereigntist subject, must have a hard body that is under control. Alterity lies in the open, flabby, impermanent body that the technology of physical fitness tries so hard to exclude. And more deeply, following my analysis from chapter 2 of puissance as the *opening* in the play of presence and absence, I suggest that this is the quintessential opening of the body through which we can appreciate its ultimately impermanent nature and deterritorialize the power of pouvoir. The essential structure of movement, which is our be-ing, is our source of alterity.

Alterity means desiring compassionately and without fear of otherness; it is the opposite of body fascism. Movement, decline, decay, death (all signs of impermanence) cease to be abject. In alteritous space there is nothing to fear. It allows one to move reflectively – to reflect through movement on the technologies of our sovereign construction in a calm, contemplative, and compassionate way, so that we can *move* beyond them. Alterity allows us to face the eschatological destiny of the world as we know it, as well as the end of ourselves and of those we love, openly, fearlessly, and non-violently.

Readers of Deleuze and Guattari will know that their programs for the deterritorialization of the self are potentially violent and dangerous. Deleuze and Guattari (1987) suggest great caution in deterritorializing experiments, recommending 'the fine art of dosages.' The postmodern–Buddhist approach is very helpful in this respect. The deterritorialization that occurs in enlightened practice is not destructive or nihilistic. The point is not to destroy the self (particle), but to live beyond it (wave). For Glass, enlightenment is compassionate desire; it is living beyond human and self in the alterity of the Body of Reality, the One Bright Pearl of impermanence. For the body, this means learning to move in a way that does not violently project onto the spatiality of movement, as does the quest for control in the technology of physical fitness. Instead it flows with the play of drawing-penetrating-absence-presence, neither destroying those forces that resist that play (the technologies of human, ego, and phallus, for instance) nor affirming them. Enlightened movement occurs in another space, as it were. Commenting on the famous *Sutra of Complete Enlightenment*, Sheng-yen (1999) speaks of moving beyond the self: 'Because birth and death and nirvana are like yesterday's dream, you should know that neither arise nor perish, neither come nor go. That which is actualized is neither gained nor lost, neither grasped nor discarded. One who truly actualizes [enlightenment] does not contrive, stop, allow things to be as they are, nor annihilate [vexations]. In the midst of actualization there is neither subject nor object. Ultimately there is neither actualization nor one who actualizes!' (26).

I suggest that this trascendent potential of which Sheng-yen speaks is present in the alteritous opening of movement, in the play of presence and absence, in which the self can disappear. In my experience this is what happens in physical activity when 'I' pay attention to the opening that movement makes rather than to myself. Those who have had this experience will know it as an awareness of timelessness, oneness, and infinite connectivity. It is the Body without Organs. And it is a potential for transcendence that is always there. It is a profound awareness that can inform our more self-oriented dimensions and make us less fearful and less subject to the dictates and nihilistic tendencies of pouvoir. Alterity, in this case, is the capacity of the modern self to be profoundly altered by its own movement.

Alteritous movement opens us to the freedom of the ultimate, which Hui-Neng (1998) has called 'the great insight having reached the other shore' (16 ff) – a Buddhist concept expressed in the Sanskrit mantra *maha-prajnaparamita*. This calls on a metaphor of crossing the sea to reach another shore: you do not destroy the original shore to get there, you simply arrive at the other shore and look back. Looking from that other shore, one can gaze on the original shore compassionately, from beyond creation and destruction. But one needs to be careful with this metaphor of another shore. For this other shore is not linearly and temporally distant from the original. Associating this with my discussion of puissance and pouvoir, we can say that reaching the other shore represents the insight that even in the making of pouvoir there is puissance, that the beyond of infinity is already there. Enlightened movement is beyond the destruction of nihilism, including the nihilistic technological destruction of the planet. The 'content' of this insight cannot be communicated in words. It is a quality that has to be moved through inwardly. As we move through the 'exteriority' of striated, finite, linear space and time – swimming the length of a pool, for example, or running through a valley, or practising tai chi – we can move into the 'interiority' of the smooth space and time of the infinite. The infinite becomes the lived reference point, the other shore, from which we can understand where we have been and where we are going, fearlessly and absolutely without aggression. In this profound appreciation of movement, of the puissance of desire, we do not need to be fearful, because the movement opens us to the empty space, the loving space, that *gives*. And with sufficient exposure to such space, we can become compassionate in our dealings with fear, anger, and the pantheon of modern exploitive and destructive strategies of which the technology of physical fitness is but one.

Notes

Introduction

1 See, for example, Bourdieu 1973; Brodeur 1988; Harvey, Beamish, and Defrance 1993; Ingham 1985; Kidd, 1996 #1072; Laberge and Sankoff 1988; and Stein 1982). On individualism and health, see Crawford 1978; 1980; Glassner 1989; Illich 1976; Krauze 1977; McKeown 1976; Powels 1973). The technology of physical fitness has been examined in its relationship to the logics of consumer culture; see Harvey and Sparks 1991; Bordo 1993; Crawford 1984; Featherstone 1991; Hoberman 1994. Some writers have been critical of the ways in which the technology of physical fitness treat the body as a machine (Hoberman 1992; 1994). Inspired by a well-known article by Donna Haraway, 'A Manifesto for Cyborgs: Science, Technology, and Socialist-Feminism in the 1980s' (Haraway 1985), some feminists have considered the potential of cyborg imagery for analysing machinic cultures of physical fitness (Balsamo 1998).

2 See, for example, Balsamo 1994; Bartky 1988; Bolin 1992; 1992; Bordo 1993; Cole 1991; 1993; 1998; Featherstone 1991; Holmlund 1994; Kidd 1987; Martin 1989; Messner 1992; Messner and Sabo 1990; 1994; Pronger 1990; Whitson 1990; 1994; Wolf 1990.

3 See, for example, Cahn 1994; Cole 1998; Lenskyj 1992; Pronger 1990; 1999a; 1999b; 2000.

4 See, for example, MacKinnon 1982; Standing Committee on Health and Welfare 1991; Whitson 1994.

5 See, for example, Bordo 1993; Hesse-Biber 1996; Spitzack 1990.

6 See, for example, Dyer 1982; Bolin 1992; 1992; Cole 1994; Connell 1987; 1990; Markula 1995; Messner 1992; Pronger 1990; Whitson 1990; 1994.

7 See, for example, Bordo 1993; Colquhoun 1990; Gleyse 1998; Harvey 1986; Harvey and Sparks 1991; Kirk and Tinning 1994; Kirk and Twigg 1994; 1995.

8 Demers 1988; MacIntosh 1986; Vertinsky 1995; 1992; 1991.

9 See Harvey 1986; Harvey, Beamish, and Defrance 1993; Kirk 1994; Kirk and Tinning 1994; Kirk and Twigg 1994; Sparks 1990.

10 Consider, for instance, the irony of Greenpeace environmentalists using high-technology communications systems to promulgate around the world their message about the perils of technology and globalization.

11 This is the oft-repeated critique of Hegel's system (Adorno 1973; Cornell 1992; Derrida 1978; 1986; Taylor 1987).

1 Theory of Science: Practice, Power, Consensus

1 Let me clarify what I mean here by 'politics.' It is a general term, as Foucault uses it, referring not necessarily to the state, bureaucracies, civil administration, and so on, but to the social discourses that influence the possibilities for daily life. This is politics in a broad sense – the politics of language, gender, sexuality, and so on. This is the political realm in which human experience is governed by social and cultural discourse.

2 The CPAFLA is a set of procedures used to evaluate specific fitness components and to recommend physical fitness regimens. These include standardized measurements of anthropometry, aerobic fitness, muscular strength, flexibility, and muscular endurance, which the test then compares to norms and percentiles of the general Canadian population. The Canadian Society for Exercise Physiology (CSEP, formerly the Canadian Association of Sport Sciences) has adopted the CPAFLA in the National Physical Fitness Appraisal Certification and Accreditation (FACA) program, which the minister for state, fitness and amateur sport mandated the CSEP to administer in 1979. The Fitness Directorate is now under the authority of Health Canada. Ability to conduct the CPAFLA is the basis for registration as a certified fitness consultant (CFC). Individuals accredited to conduct more advanced fitness protocols become certified fitness appraisers. The CPAFLA is, within the exercise science establishment, a highly credentiallized work of scientific technology.

3 There are other, more 'accurate' tests of specific parameters of fitness, such as 'maximal oxygen uptake' testing with metabolic analysis and hydrostatic weighing for estimating fat content. These more 'accurate'

tests, complex and expensive, are much more rare than tests such as the CPAFLA, which is routine in recreation centres and fitness clubs. My university department's physical fitness testing facility uses the CPAFLA.

4 WHO's definition of health promotion is 'the process of enabling individuals and communities to increase control over and to improve their health' (World Health Organization 1984, 3).

5 I use 'government' with a lower-case 'g' to refer to government in Foucault's sense. Where I am referring to government in the sense of the government of Canada, I use 'government' with its domain – for example, Canadian government, Ontario government.

6 The *Canadian Standardized Test of Fitness Interpretation and Counselling Manual* (Canadian Association of Sport Sciences 1987a, 142) lists a number of similar texts as reference sources. Most chapters in the *American College of Sports Medicine's Resource Guidelines for Exercise Testing and Prescription* (ACSM 1993) cite similar texts.

7 On the rhetoric of scientific citation of texts – as it were, the intertextuality of scientific texts – see Latour 1987, 30–44). I develop this theme in my deconstructive analysis of the texts of fitness testing in chapter 3.

8 This involves not only a complex textual rhetoric, but also a good deal of political manoeuvring among scientists in the process of getting published (deciding who is part of the research team, first authorship, and so on), as well as the prestige of the scientists involved – I discuss this point more fully in the following paragraphs. Moreover, because experiments are profoundly intertextual, no one actually ever 'sees' the experiment fully.

9 This is far from a static situation. There are frequent political struggles over what kind of thinking will be dominant and where to draw boundaries. And changes in the guard do occur. New ways of thinking and new boundaries become established. This fact points to the truly political nature of journals.

10 While he does not make overt political connections regarding how science hides its social nature, Latour refers to this practice as 'black boxing,' which, for the sake of simplicity, hides the social complexity of the construction of scientific facts.

2 Theory of the Body: Technology, Puissance, and Pouvoir

1 For more thorough reviews of socio-cultural theories of the body, see Featherstone, Hepworth, and Turner 1991; Shilling 1993; Turner 1984; 1991; 1992; 1997.

2 Karl Marx 1964, of course, has also expressed outrage over this state of affairs, which resonates throughout the work of his many critical inheritors.

3 Cf Heidegger on the meaning of 'responsibility' (Heidegger 1954, 290–2).

4 Historically, these philosophical debates, at least as they reach us in texts, have been conducted by men and completely excluded women. Women too can share in this domineering subjectivity. Indeed, Donna Haraway resents the notion that women are somehow essentially environmentally connected 'earth mothers.'

5 Though Massumi points out that they do not always observe the terminological difference.

6 Because these words appear frequently in the remainder of this book, and in order to render them less 'exotic,' I anglicize them and do not place them in italics.

7 The *Oxford English Dictionary* defines energy as an 'exercise of power, actual working, operation, activity.'

8 Although imperialism goes to work by taking hold of the essence of beings, pouvoir, as I argue at length below, seizes on puissance (essence), thus producing itself.

9 Massumi (1992) points out: 'In numerous passages in many of his works, Deleuze rejects the term "essence" because of its Platonic overtones, preferring such terms as "event," "problem," "Aion," or "Idea"' (148 n20). Heidegger's concept of essence as coming to presence is an event, as I show below.

10 Heidegger, not fancying himself a political philosopher (his apparent silence on his own Nazism proving this point all too emphatically), did not thematize extensively the political psychology of controlling being. But the hypostatization about which Sheehan (1981) speaks is a way of controlling being.

11 There are only two passing references to Heidegger in *A Thousand Plateaus* (125 and 561 n85) and none in *Anti-Oedipus*.

12 I distilled the reflections below on the body, movement, and being from several sources. They are inspired particularly by the later writings of Heidegger, especially his thoughts on *Ereignis* as the eventfulness of being (Heidegger 1972). I also draw on thoughts from my MSc thesis (Pronger 1991) and my PhD thesis (Pronger 1996), an article on postmodernism and science (Pronger 1995), an article on postmodernism and sport (Pronger 1998), and others (Pronger 1990; 1991; 1992; 1994; 1995).

13 For the primacy of the Western gaze in the canonical authors of queer theory, for instance, see de Lauretis 1991; Duberman 1997; Golding 1997;

Morton 1996; Probyn 1995; Seidman 1993; Simpson 1996; Sinfield 1994; Warner 1993. Most of the authors to whom I allude in this book exclude non-Western intellectual traditions from their work. Some notable exceptions are Glass 1995; Levin 1987; 1985; Lingis 1983; Martin 1992; Parkes 1987; Stambaugh, 1999 #1457; 1990; Warren 1994.

14 See Edward Said on the colonialism of the exclusionary structure of the East–West distinction (Said 1978 [1994]).

15 I am referring here to sexualities that have their cultural basis in the power relations of the gender myth. I explore this theme in chapter 2 of my book (Pronger 1992).

16 It is a deeply patriarchal assumption that only men can penetrate. For this assumes that penetration is accomplished first and foremost by a phallus. But it is heterosexist and phallocentric to assume that the phallus is the only thing that can penetrate or, indeed, that the vagina is the only orifice for penetration.

17 Paraphrasing Heidegger on this point, Sheehan (1981) says: 'The presence-of-its-absentiality (or its privative presence) is the moving entitiy's being-structure. We may call it "pres-ab-sentiality"' (537).

18 Glass's account of the three readings of emptiness is complex and nuanced. Unfortunately, I cannot render the sophistication of his arguments here. I mention the first two readings only to give a sense of the contrast that the third represents.

19 My use of the word 'eros' is not in any way related to Freud's concept for the entire complex of life-preservative instincts. Freud's theory of instincts serves a functional logic of the human psyche. Understanding human being primarily in terms of function, I argue below, is an epistemic strategy of pouvoir. In Deleuze's terms, it is part of the knowledge-based organization of the body that blocks/channels the free flow of desire. In Foucault's terms, it is a knowing, inscribing, circumscribing gaze that establishes power (pouvoir) over the body (which, for Foucault, includes mind/psyche) by determining its proper uses.

20 In this conception of power, Foucault is speaking of the historical construction of power as a relation. As such, power circulates in various forms, which he calls discourses. Such discourses can include gender, race, and sexuality. Modern power is characterized not by a particular discourse, but by the (characteristic) ways in which discourse(s) are operationalized.

21 Anyone with intense athletic experience knows that pleasure is only one way of looking at the pain of extreme exertion.

22 In a paper presented at the 1993 meeting of the North American Society

for the Sociology of Sport, Suzanne Laberge argued that Bourdieu's theory of physical capital can be expanded beyond class to include gender.

23 Massumi (1992) defines 'socius' as follows: 'A society is a dissipative structure with its own determining tension between a limitive body without organs [pouvoir] and a nonlimitive one [puissance]. Together, in their interaction, they are called a "socius" (the abstract machine of society)' (75).

24 A complete discussion here of Deleuze and Guattari's voluminous theory and history of the relations of desire and capitalism is impossible. I am borrowing from them only some basic analytical 'tools' (Massumi 1992, 8).

25 This is not to say that religion or psychiatry is chronologically exclusive of capitalism. Obviously, religious influence continues under capitalism, but to a lesser and lesser degree and on more and more capitalist terms. Christianity and Judaism especially have been influenced by (capitalist) modernization. Psychiatry is modernized religion. Religious and psychiatric codes 'return' in capitalism as part of the recodification of desire that reins in its freedom.

26 This dichotomy between extrinsic and intrinsic should not be confused with external and internal systems of power, as Foucault has contrasted pre-modern and modern political systems of control. I am suggesting that an extrinsic meaning structure (use-value to a social, political, economic system) becomes internalized and charts the course of the body's power of movement, displacing its intrinsic freedom.

27 But in this argument that bodies/desires are produced as resources for the economic system, how do we account for the growing underclass, the mass of desire that is underused in this system in terms of both production and consumption? Capitalism has refined its human resource base so well, is producing it to be so efficient, that most people become waste products, detritus next to fewer and fewer perfectly productive bodies. There is an analogy here to nuclear energy, which is the most intensive exploitation of a resource, getting the most energy out of the least material. Likewise we now have the technology to get the most work out of the fewest people, the ultimate exploitation. And just as in nuclear energy vast waste and destruction occur in its production, so to the high technology of human resources produces vast human waste in the form of an ever-growing underclass, both within 'developed' countries and even more extensively in the vastly impoverished 'third,' or 'developing' world. And the enthusiasm of new right governments to cut even the most rudimentary support for the underclasses is testimony to their status

as detritus. In this economy of bodies and desire, then, it becomes imperative for individuals to capitalize on the economic utility of their desire maximally, to compete with each other in the marketplace of producing consuming desire if they are to be part of the system at all.
28 The extent to which race and gender contribute to the resourcing/wasting of the body/desire in the technology of physical fitness I examine in chapter 3.

3 The Texts of the Technology of Physical Fitness

1 'Healthy Cities' is a category of health promotion for the WHO.
2 In 1998, AIDS appeared as a subject 3,640 times, roughly half the number of citations as for exercise. From 1966 to 1998, cancer appeared as a subject 258,632 times, a little more than twice the frequency of exercise.
3 Most departments also offer activity courses where students learn various mainstream Euro–American sports and training methods. Very few offer activity courses on non-hegemonic sports, games, and activities, such as tai chi, yoga, pilates, body awareness, bocci, and kabadi. And there are many kinesiology and physical education departments that focus not so much on the technology of health as on the technology of competitive, high-performance sport, which is not my main concern in this book.
4 This is not to say that the entire experience of exercise is reduced to that interpretive framework. In some instances, 'progress' in exercise and charting that 'progress' are essential to the enterprise. In others, measurement is more of a ritual structure for other dimensions of the moving body.
5 The Fédération internationale de Volleyball, as part of its marketing scheme, for instance, requires *women* athletes to wear skimpy outfits that display their bodies by using minimal amounts of material and fabrics such as lycra that adhere closely to the body – they may not wear loose clothing. Not having yet tapped into such frank erotic marketing for male athletes, they do not require the same of men.

4 Writing the Fascist Body: Description, Inscription, Prescription

1 One of the great breakthroughs of modern scientific technological hermeneutics was to understand the human body as essentially no different from any other body. This was a major departure from traditional Aristotelian physics, which understood different bodies as having essentially different natures. Heidegger (1977) believes that Newton

articulated this modern *logos* in his first law of motion: 'Every body continues in its state of rest, or uniform motion in a straight line, unless it is compelled to change that state by force impressed upon it' (256). For Heidegger, the reductionism of Newton's '*every* body' marks the violence of Newton's (and modernity's) conceptual universe. This standardization of the hermeneutics of the real gave technological humans vast power over the real: no deference need be paid to essential differences. This 'every body' expresses what Mark Taylor has identified as one of the hallmarks of modernity: the enclosure of difference. Everything, when treated as essentially the same in physical terms, becomes available to technological manipulation. Recent advances in genetic technology and the patenting of genomes highlight the cultural complexity of this fundamental technological hermeneutics.

2 The few who do so tend to explore the experience of flow and transcendent feelings that can come from intense (usually prolonged) exercise. While there are interesting texts on this matter – most published in the 1970s, when universities' physical education departments had significant complements of philosophers and other 'arts'-oriented scholars – the more recent techno-scientization of physical education has rendered this work entirely marginal. Those academic exercise sciences interested in the 'experience' of physical activity study it in terms of psychopharmacology, an entirely anthropocentric undertaking. The now-popular reductionist notion that such experiences are caused by the release of endorphins – which are 'natural' pain *killers* – is the product of this kind of domineering knowledge-production.

3 The probable collapse of the ecosphere, brought about by the technological domination of Man, would mark the failure of sovereign domination by modern Man.

4 See my discussions of paradigms above in chapter 1.

5 As I argue below, popular representations of the fit body reproduce the reality of the laboratory, in so far as they themselves use the iconographic *products* of the scientific technology of physical fitness.

6 Texts of the third circle can also be texts of the first. For instance, someone undergoing a fitness test in a commercial gym may have already done some of the tests available on the worldwide web and in the popular texts of physical fitness. Familiarity with fitness testing in its different formats and with reading one's own body through the texts of testing contribute to the ambient textuality.

7 As I show below, people do contribute significantly to the narratives produced in the first circle of texts, but only within the logos of the

technology of physical fitness, unless they are able to reject that logos – a possibility that the circles of texts try to prevent.

8 The mirror comparison that I have said works as a confessional continues to rely on the subjectivity of the 'penitent' and as such may be more or less compromising in its accusations.

9 There is a parallel in financial capital to this discourse on accumulation of physical capital: 'You may have money now, but you better save for emergencies and your old age.'

10 Howard Stein (1982) says: 'The fitness-wellness-health ethos is further part of the anti-intellectual (or psuedo-intellectual) attitude that substitutes insight with action' (169).

Bibliography

Abram, David. 1983. 'Natural Magic.' *Minding the Earth: Newsletter of the Strong Centre for Environmental Values* 4 (2).

Adorno, Theodor. 1973. *Negative Dialectics*. Trans. E.B. Ashton. New York: Continuum.

Adorno, Theodor, and Max Horkheimer. 1972. *Dialectic of Enlightenment*. Trans. J. Cumming. New York: Herder and Herder.

Alderman, Harold. 1978. 'Heidegger's Critique of Modern Science and Technology.' In M. Murray, ed., *Heidegger and Modern Philosophy*, 35–50. New Haven, Conn.: Yale University Press.

Allman, Fred. 1994. 'Forty Years of Progress: Surgical Approach to Care of Injured Athletes.' In *Fortieth Anniversary Lectures*, ed. American College of Sports Medicine. Indianapolis: American College of Sports Medicine.

Althuser, Louis. 1977. 'Ideology and Ideological State Apparatuses (Notes towards an Investigation).' In *Lenin and Philosophy and Other Essays*. London: New Left Books.

American College of Sports Medicine (ACSM). 1993. *American College of Sports Medicine's Resource Guidelines for Exercise Testing and Prescription*. Philadelphia: Lea & Febiger.

– 1994. *Fortieth Anniversary Lectures*. Indianapolis: American College of Sports Medicine.

Arendt, Hannah. 1968. *The Origins of Totalitarianism*. New York: Harcourt Brace and World.

Ashcroft, Bill, Gareth Griffiths, and Helen Tiffin, eds. 1995. *The Post-colonial Studies Reader*. London: Routledge.

Bain, Linda. 1990. 'A Critical Analysis of the Hidden Curriculum in Physical Education.' In D. Kirk and R. Tinning, eds., *Physical Education, Curriculum and Culture: Critical Issues in the Contemporary Crisis*. New York: Falmer Press.

Balsamo, A. 1994. 'Feminist Body-building.' In S. Birrell and C. Cole, eds., *Women, Sport and Culture*. Urbana-Champagne, Ill: Human Kinetics Press.

Balsamo, Anne. 1998. *Technologies of the Gendered Body: Reading Cyborg Women*. Durham, NC: Duke University Press.

Barsky, Robert. 1993. 'Discourse Analysis Theory.' In I. Makaryk, ed., *Encyclopedia of Contemporary Literary Theory: Approaches, Scholars, Terms*. Toronto: University of Toronto Press.

Bartky, Sandra Lee. 1988. 'Foucault, Femininity, and the Modernization of Patriarchal Power. In I. Diamond and L. Quinby, eds., *Feminism and Foucault*. Boston: Northeastern University Press.

Bataille, Georges. 1977. *Death and Sensuality: A Study of Eroticism and the Taboo*. New York: Arno.

– 1986. *Eroticism: Death and Sensuality*. San Francisco: City Lights.

– 1988. *Inner Experience*. Trans. L.A. Boldt. Buffalo: SUNY Press.

– n.d. *Lascaux, or the Birth of Art*. Trans. A. Wainhouse. Switzerland: Kira.

Bauman, Zygmunt. 1998. 'Postmodern Religion?' In P. Heelas, ed., In *Religion, Modernity and Postmodernity*. Oxford: Blackwell.

Bazerman, Charles. 1988. *Shaping Written Knowledge: The Genre and Activity of the Experimental Article in Science*. Madison: University of Wisconsin Press.

Beamish, Robert. 1982. 'Some Neglected Political Themes in Sport Study.' Paper read to The American Sociological Association, San Francisco.

Beck, Ulrich. 1992. *Risk Society: Towards a New Modernity*. London: Sage.

Bell, Rudolph M. 1985. *Holy Anorexia*. Chicago: University of Chicago Press.

Bercovitz, Kim. 1996. 'A Critical Analysis of Canada's "Active Living": Science or Politics?' Doctoral thesis, Community Health, University of Toronto, Toronto.

Berry, Thomas. 1988. *The Dream of the Earth*. San Francisco: Sierra Club Books.

Bleier, Ruth. 1984. *Science and Gender: A Critique of Biology and Its Theories on Women*. New York: Pergamon Press.

Bolin, Ann. 1992a. 'Beauty or Beast: The Subversive Soma.' In C.B. Cohen, ed., *Body Contours: Deciphering Scripts of Gender and Power*. New Brunswick, NJ: Rutgers University Press.

– 1992b. 'Flex Appeal, Food and Fat: Competitive Bodybuilding, Gender and Diet.' *Play and Culture* 5: 378–400.

– 1992c. 'Vandalized Vanity: Feminine Physiques Betrayed and Portrayed.' In F. Mascia-Lees, ed., *Tattoo, Torture, Adornment and Disfigurement: The Denaturalization of the Body in Culture and Text*. Albany: State University of New York Press.

Bordo, S. 1990. 'Reading the Slender Body.' In Jacobus, Fox-Keller, and Shuttleworth, eds., *Body Politics*.

Bordo, Susana. 1993a. 'Reading the Male Body.' *Michigan Quarterly Review* 32 (fall): 696–737.

– 1993b. *Unbearable Weight: Feminism, Western Culture and the Body*. Berkeley: University of California Press.

– 1999. *The Male Body: A New Look at Men in Public and Private*. New York: Farrar, Straus and Giroux.

Bouchard, Claude, Roy J. Shephard, and Thomas Stephens. 1992. *Physical Activity, Fitness, and Health: International Proceedings and Consensus Statement, International Conference on Physical Activity, Fitness and Health*. Toronto: Human Kinetics.

Bourdieu, Pierre. 1973. 'Cultural Reproduction and Social Reproduction.' In R. Brown, ed., *Knowledge, Education and Social Change*. London: Tavistock.

– 1978. 'Sport and Social Class.' *Social Science Information* 17: 819–40.

– 1979. 'Symbolic Power.' *Critique of Anthropology* 4 (summer): 77–85.

– 1984. *Distinction: A Social Critique of the Judgement of Taste*. London: Routledge.

– 1988a. 'The Forms of Capital.' In J. Richardson, ed., *Handbook of Theory and Research in Education*. New York: Greenwood Press.

– 1988b. 'Program for a Sociology of Sport.' *Sociology of Sport Journal* 5 (2): 153–61.

– 1990. *The Logic of Practice*. Stanford, Calif.: Stanford University.

Bourdieu, Pierre, and Jean-Claude Passeron. 1990. *Reproduction in Education, Society and Culture*. Trans. R. Nice, ed. M. Featherstone. *Theory, Culture & Society*. London: Sage.

Brodeur, Pierre. 1988. 'Employee Fitness: Doctrines and Issues.' In J. Harvey and H. Cantelon, eds., *Not Just a Game: Essays in Canadian Sport Sociology*. Ottawa: University of Ottawa Press.

Brooks, George. 1994. 'Basic Exercise Physiology.' In ACSM 1994.

Brungardt, Kurt, Brett Brungardt, and Mike Brungardt. 1995. *The Complete Book of Butt and Legs: Over One Hundred Exercises [and] Dozens of Routines for Home and Gym. Get the Best Results in the Shortest Time*. New York: Villard Books.

Butler, Judith. 1990. *Gender Trouble: Feminism and the Subversion of Identity*. New York: Routledge.

Cahn, Susan K. 1994. *Coming on Strong: Gender and Sexuality in Twentieth-Century Women's Sport*. Cambridge, Mass.: Harvard University Press.

Callari, Antonio, Stephen Cullenberg, and Carole Biewener, eds. 1995. *Marxism in the Postmodern Age: Confronting the New World Order*. New York: Guilford Press.

Cambell, Murray. 2001. 'Cheney's Plan on Blackouts: Get More Fuel.' *Globe and Mail*, 1 May 2001, A12.

Canada. 1969. *Task Force Reports on the Costs of Health Services in Canada*. Ottawa: Queen's Printer.

– 1972. *Proceedings of the National Conference on Fitness and Health*. Ottawa: National Health and Welfare.

– 1973. *The Community Health Centre in Canada*. Ottawa: Information Canada.

Canadian Association of Sport Sciences. 1987a. *Canadian Standardized Test of Fitness Interpretation and Counselling Manual*. Gloucester, Ont.: Canadian Association of Sport Sciences.

– 1987b. *Canadian Standardized Test of Fitness Operations Manual*. 3rd ed. Gloucester, Ont.: Canadian Association of Sport Sciences.

Canadian Fitness and Lifestyle Research Institute: *Warning to Couch Potatoes*. 9 Feb. 2002. Available from http://www.cflri.ca/cflri/tips/98/LT98_01.html

Canadian Society for Exercise Physiology (CSEP). 1996. *The Canadian Physical Activity, Fitness and Lifestyle Appraisal: CSEP's Plan for Healthy Active Living*. 2nd ed. Ottawa: Canadian Society for Exercise Physiology.

Caputo, John D. 1986. *The Mystical Element in Heidegger's Thought*. New York: Fordham University Press.

Carroll, John. 1993. *Humanism: The Wreck of Western Culture*. London: Fontana.

Champagne, John. 1995. *The Ethics of Marginality*. Minneapolis: University of Minnesota Press.

Chardin, Teilhard de. 1959. *The Phenomenon of Man*. Trans. B. Wall. New York: Harper.

Charles, John M. 1998. 'Technology and the Body.' *Quest* 50 (4): 379–88.

Cole, Cheryl. 1991. 'The Politics of Cultural Representation: Visions of Fields/ Fields of Visions.' *International Review of the Sociology of Sport* 26 (1): 37–52.

– 1993. 'Resisting the Canon: Feminist Cultural Studies, Sport and Technologies of the Body.' *Journal of Sport and Social Issues* 17 (2): 77–97.

– 1994. 'Theorizing Sociology in the Age of Sexuality.' Paper read to the Pacific Sociological Association, San Diego.

– 1998. 'Addiction, Exercise, and Cyborgs: Technologies of Deviant Bodies.' In G. Rail, ed., *Sport and Postmodern Times*, Buffalo: SUNY Press.

Colquhoun, Derek. 1990. 'Images of Healthism in Health-Based Physical Education.' In D. Kirk and R. Tinning, eds., *Physical Education, Curriculum and Culture: Critical Issues in the Contemporary Crisis*. New York: Falmer Press.

Comay, Rebecca. 1995. Introduction. *Alphabet City: Fascism and Its Ghosts*. Vol. 4–5 combined: 2–3.

Connell, Robert. 1987. *Gender and Power: Society, the Person and Sexual Politics*. Cambridge: Polity.

– 1990. 'An Iron Man: The Body and Some Contradictions of Hegemonic Masculinity.' In M. Messner and D. Sabo, eds., *Sport, Men and the Gender Order*. Champaign, Ill.: Human Kinetics.

Cook, Francis. 1977. *Hua-yen Buddhism: The Jewel Net of Indra*. University Park: Pennsylvania State University Press.

Cooper, Kenneth. 1982. *The Aerobics Program for Total Well-Being*. New York: M. Evans and Co.

Cornell, Drucilla. 1992. *The Philosophy of the Limit*. New York: Routledge.

Costill, David, Ernest Maglischo, and Allen Richardson. 1992. *Swimming*. Oxford: Blackwell Scientific Publications.

Crawford, Robert. 1978. 'You Are Dangerous to Your Health.' *Social Policy* (Jan./Feb.): 11–20.

– 1980. 'Healthism and the Medicalization of Everyday Life.' *International Journal of Health Services* 10 (3): 365–88.

– 1984. 'A Cultural Account of "Health": Control, Release. and the Social Body.' In J. B. McKinlay, ed., *Issues in the Political Economy of Health Care*. New York: Tavistock.

Crawford, Trish. 1995. 'Survival of the Fittest.' *Toronto Star*, 24 Sept., D6, D5.

Critchley, Simon. 1992. *The Ethics of Deconstruction: Derrida and Levinas*. Cambridge, Mass.: Oxford University Press.

Davis, M., P. Fanning, and M. McKay. 1983. *The Communications Book*. Oakland, Calif.: New Harksinger Publications.

de Lauretis, Teresa, ed. 1991. *Queer Theory. A Special Edition of Differences* 3(2): i–xviii, 1–159.

Deleuze, Gilles. 1992. 'Postscript on the Societies of Control.' *October* 59 (winter): 3–7.

Deleuze, Gilles, and Felix Guattari. 1983. *Anti-Oedipus: Capitalism and Schizophrenia*. Trans. R. Hurley, M. Seem, and H.L. Lane. Minneapolis: University of Minnesota Press.

– 1987. *A Thousand Plateaus: Capitalism and Schizophrenia*. Trans. B. Massumi. Minneapolis: University of Minnesota Press.

Delumeau, Jean. 1990. *Sin and Fear: The Emergence of Western Guilt Culture, 13th–18th Centuries*. New York: St Martin's Press.

Demers, Pierre. 1988. 'University Training of Physical Educators.' In J. Harvey and H. Cantelon, eds., *Not Just a Game: Essays in Canadian Sport Sociology*. Ottawa: University of Ottawa Press.

Derrida, Jacques. 1978. *Writing and Difference*. Trans. A. Bass. Chicago: University of Chicago Press.

– 1986. *Glas*. Trans. by J.P. Leavey Jr, and R. Rand. Lincoln: University of Nebraska University Press.

– 1987. *The Truth in Painting*. Trans. by G. Bennington and I. McLeod. Chicago: University of Chicago Press.

Dews, Peter. 1987. *Logics of Disintegration: Post-structuralist Thought and the Claims of Critical Theory*. London: Verso.

Dillard, Annie. 1982. 'Teaching a Stone to Talk.' In Gotlieb 1996.

– 1999. *For the Time Being*. Toronto: Penguin.

Doan, Laura, ed. 1994. *The Lesbian Postmodern*. New York: Columbia University Press.

Dreyfus, Hubert, and Paul Rabinow. 1983. *Michel Foucault: Beyond Structuralism and Hermeneutics*. 2nd ed. Chicago: University of Chicago Press.

Duberman, Martin, ed. 1997. *A Queer World: The Center for Lesbian and Gay Studies Reader*. New York: New York University Press.

Dyer, Ken. 1982. *Challenging the Men: The Social Biology of Female Sporting Achievement*. St Lucia: University of Queensland Press.

Dyer, Richard. 1997. *White*. London: Routledge.

Ebert, Teresa. 1996. *Ludic Feminism and After: Postmodernism, Desire, and Labor in Late Capitalism, Critical Perspectives on Women and Gender*. Ann Arbor: University of Michigan Press.

Egan, G. 1975. *The Skilled Helper*. Monterey, Calif.: Brooks/Cole.

Falk, Pasi. 1994. *The Consuming Body, Theory, Culture, and Society*. London: Sage.

Farley, Kara Leverte, and Sheil M. Curry. 1994. *Get Motivated! Daily Psych-Ups: Whether You Work Out, Play Weekend Sports or Compete Professionally, This Book Will Get You Started and Keep You Going*. New York: Fireside.

Fay, B. 1987. *Critical Social Science*. Ithaca, NY: Cornell University Press.

Featherstone, Mike. 1991. 'The Body in Consumer Culture.' In Featherstone, Hepworth, and Turner 1991.

Featherstone, Mike, Mike Hepworth, and Bryan S. Turner, eds. 1991. *The Body: Social Process and Cultural Theory*. London: Sage.

Fitness Ontario. 1984. *Sticking with Fitness*. Toronto: Ontario Ministry of Tourism and Recreation.

Foltz, Bruce. 1995. *Inhabiting the Earth: Heidegger, Environmental Ethics, and the Metphysics of Nature*. Atlantic Heights, NJ: Humanities Press.

Foucault, Michel. 1975. *The Birth of the Clinic: An Archaeology of Medical Perception*. Trans. A.M.S. Smith, ed. R.D. Laing. New York: Vintage.

– 1979. *Discipline and Punish: The Birth of the Prison*. Trans. by A. Sheridan. New York: Vintage.

– 1980a. *The History of Sexuality: Volume I: An Introduction*. Trans. R. Hurley. Vol. I. New York: Vintage.

- 1980b. *Power/Knowledge: Selected Interviews and Other Writings 1972–1977*. Trans. C. Gordon, L. Marshall, J. Mepham, and K. Soper. New York: Pantheon.
- 1981. 'The Order of Discourse.' In R. Young, ed., *Untying the Text: A Post-structuralist Reader*. Boston: Routledge.
- 1983a. 'Preface.' In Deleuze and Grattain, *Anti-Oedipus: Capitalism and Schizophrenia*. Minneapolis: University of Minnesota Press.
- 1983b. 'The Subject and Power.' In Dreyfus and Rabinow 1983.
- 1988. 'Technologies of the Self.' In L. Martin, H. Gutman, and P. Hutton, eds., *Technologies of the Self: A Seminar with Michel Foucault*. Amherst: University of Massachusetts Press.

Friel, Joe. 1998. *The Triathlete's Training Bible: A Complete Training Guide for the Competitive Multisport Athlete*. Boulder, Col.: Velo.

Fusco, Caroline. In progress. 'A Social Theory of Locker Room Spaces.' PhD thesis, Exercise Science, University of Toronto, Toronto.

Game, Ann. 1991. *Undoing the Social: Towards a Deconstructive Sociology*. Toronto: University of Toronto Press.

Ginzberg, Ruth. 1989. 'Uncovering Gynocentric Science.' In N. Tuana, ed., *Feminism and Science*. Bloomington: Indiana University Press.

Gladwell, Malcolm. 1997. 'The Sports Taboo: Why Blacks Are Like Boys and Whites Are Like Girls.' *New Yorker*, 19 May 1997.

Glass, Robert Newman. 1995. *Working Emptiness: Toward a Third Reading of Emptiness in Buddhism and Postmodern Thought*. Atlanta: Scholars Press.

Glassner, Barry. 1989. 'Fitness and the Postmodern Self.' *Journal of Health and Social Behavior* 30 (June): 180–91.

Glazebrook, Trish. In press. 'Heidegger and Ecofeminism.' In P. Huntington and N. Holland, eds., *Feminist Interpretations of Martin Heidegger*. University Park: Pennsylvania State University Press.

Gleyse, Jacques. 1998. 'Instrumental Rationalization of Human Movement: An Archeological Approach.' In G. Rail, ed., *Sport and Postmodern Times*. Buffalo: SUNY Press.

Goldberg, David Theo. 1993. *Racist Culture: Philosophy and the Politics of Meaning*. Oxford: Blackwell.
- ed. 1990. *Anatomy of Racism*. Minneapolis: University of Minnesota Press.

Golding, Sue. 1997. *The Eight Technologies of Otherness*. New York: Routledge.

Gorer, Geoffrey. 1965. *Death, Grief and Mourning in Contemporary Britain*. London: Cresset Press.

Gottlieb, Roger S., ed. 1996. *This Sacred Earth: Religion, Nature, Environment*. New York: Routledge.

Grace, Victoria. 1991. 'The Marketing of Empowerment and the Construction of the Health Consumer: A Critique of Health Promotion.' *International Journal of Health Services* 21 (2): 329–43.

Gray, Chris Hables, ed. 1995. *The Cyborg Handbook*. New York: Routledge.

Greenspon, Edward. 1996. 'Economy Changing Far Faster Than People.' *Globe and Mail*, 20 Apr., A1, A12–13.

Grosz, Elizabeth. 1995. *Space, Time and Perversion*. New York: Routledge.

Grosz, Elizabeth, and Elspeth Probyn, eds. 1995. *Sexy Bodies: The Strange Carnalities of Feminism*. New York: Routledge.

Habermas, Jurgen. 1983. 'Modernity: An Incomplete Project.' In H. Foster, ed., *The Anti-aesthetic: Essays on Postmodern Culture*. Port Townsend, Wash.: Bay Press.

Hacking, Ian. 1992. 'Making People Up.' In E. Stein, ed., *Forms of Desire: Sexual Orientation and the Social Construction Controversy*. New York: Routledge.

– 1995. 'The Looping Effects of Human Kinds.' In D. Serber, D. Premack, and A. Premack, eds., *Causal Cognition: An Interdisciplinary Approach*. Oxford: Oxford University Press.

Hall, S., C. Critcher, T. Jefferson, J. Clarke, and B. Roberts. 1978. *Policing the Crisis: Mugging, the State and Law and Order*. Houndmills: Macmillan.

Haraway, Donna. 1985. 'A Manifesto for Cyborgs: Science, Technology, and Socialist-Feminism in the 1980s.' *Socialist Review* 80: 65–107.

– 1988. 'Situated Knowledges: The Science Question in Feminism and the Privilege of Partial Perspective.' *Feminist Studies* 3 (fall): 575–99.

Harding, Sandra. 1986. *The Science Question in Feminism*. Ithaca, NY: Cornell University Press.

Harvey, Jean. 1983. *Le corps programmé ou la rhétorique de Kino-Québec*. Montreal: Albert Saint-Martin.

Harvey, [Jean], and R. Sparks. 1991. 'The Politics of the Body in the Context of Modernity.' *Quest* 43: 164–89.

– 1986. 'The Rationalization of Bodily Practices.' *Arena Review* 10: 55–65.

– 1988. 'Sport Policy and the Welfare State: An Outline of the Canadian Case.' *Sociology of Sport Journal* 5: 315–29.

Harvey, Jean, Bob Beamish, and Jacques Defrance. 1993. 'Physical Exercise Policy and the Welfare State: A Framework for Comparative Analysis.' *International Review for the Sociology of Sport* 28 (1): 53–63.

Hay, James, and J. Gavin Reid. 1982. *The Anatomical and Mechanical Bases of Human Motion*. Englewood Cliffs, NJ: Prentice-Hall.

Health Canada and Canadian Society for Exercise Physiology. n.d. *Handbook for Canada's Physical Activity Guide*. Ottawa: Publications Health Canada.

Heidegger, Martin. 1927. *Being and Time*. Trans. J. Macquarrie and E. Robinson. New York: Harper and Row.

– 1938. 'The Age of the World Picture.' In *The Question Concerning Technology and Other Essays*. New York: Garland.

– 1953. 'Science and Reflection.' In *The Question Concerning Technology: Heidegger's Critique of the Modern Age*. New York: Garland.

– 1954a. 'Building, Dwelling, Thinking.' In Krell 1977.

– 1954b. 'The Question Concerning Technology.' In Krell 1977b.

– 1954. 'What Calls for Thinking?' In Krell 1977b.

– 1961. 'On the Essence of Truth.' In Krell 1977b.

– 1962. 'Modern Science, Metaphysics, and Mathematics.' In Krell 1977b.

– 1966a. *Discourse on Thinking*. Trans. J.M. Anderson and E.H. Freund. New York: Harper and Row.

– 1966b. 'The End of Philosophy and the Task of Thinking.' In Krell 1977b.

– 1971. *Poetry, Language, Thought*. Trans. A. Hofstadter. New York: Harper and Row.

– 1972. *On Time and Being*. Trans. J. Stambaugh. 1st ed. New York: Harper and Row.

– 1975. 'Logos.' In *Early Greek Thinking*. San Francisco: Harper and Row.

– 1977. *The Question Concerning Technology and Other Essays*. Trans. W. Lovitt. New York: Harper and Row.

Hesse-Biber, Sharlene. 1996. *Am I Thin Enough Yet? The Cult of Thinness and the Commercialization of Identity*. New York: Oxford University Press.

Hoberman, John. 1984. *Sport and Political Ideology*. Austin: University of Texas Press.

– 1992. *Mortal Engines: The Science of Performance and the Dehumanization of Sport*. New York: Free Press.

– 1994. 'The Sportive-Dynamic Body as a Symbol of Productivity.' In T. Sioebers, *Heterotopia: Postmodern Utopia and the Body Politic*. Ann Arbor: University of Michigan Press.

Hocquenghem, Guy. 1995. 'To Destroy Sexuality.' In F. Peraldi, ed., *Polysexuality*. New York: Semiotext(e).

Hodge, John L. 1990. 'Equality: Beyond Dualism and Oppression.' In D.T. Goldberg, ed., *Anatomy of Racism*. Minneapolis: University of Minnesota Press.

Holmlund, Christine Anne. 1994. 'Visible Difference and Flex Appeal: The Body, Sex, Sexuality, and Race in the Pumping Iron Films.' In S. Birrell and C.L. Cole, eds., *Women, Sport, and Culture*. Champaign, Ill: Human Kinetics.

Honeth, Axel. 1993. 'Frankfurt School.' In W. Outhwaite and T. Bottomore, eds., *The Blackwell Dictionary of Twentieth-Century Social Thought*. Oxford: Blackwell.

hooks, bell. 1992. *Black Looks: Race and Representation*. Boston: South End Press.

– 1994. *Teaching to Transgress: Education as the Practice of Freedom*. New York: Routledge.

Horkheimer, Max, and Theodor Adorno. 1972. *Dialectic of Enlightenment*. Trans. J. Cumming. New York: Continuum.

Hubbard, Ruth. 1989. 'Science, Facts and Feminism.' In N. Tuana, ed., *Science and Feminism*. Bloomington: Indiana University Press.

– 1990. *The Politics of Women's Biology*. New Brunswick, NJ: Rutgers University Press.

Hui-Neng. 1998. *The Sutra of Hui-Neng, Grand Master of Zen*. Trans. T. Cleary. Boston: Shambhala.

Hutcheon, Linda. 1989. *The Politics of Postmodernism*. London: Routledge.

Huyssen, Andreas. 1986. *After the Great Divide: Modernism, Mass Culture, Postmodernism*. Bloomington: Indianna University Press.

Illich, Ivan. 1976. *Limits to Medicine: Medical Nemesis: The Expropriation of Health*. London: Marion Boyars.

Ingham, Alan. 1985. 'From Public Issues to Personal Trouble: Well-being and the Fiscal Crisis of the State.' *Sociology of Sport Journal* 2 (1): 43–55.

Jameson, Frederic. 1984. 'Postmodernism, or the Cultural Logic of Late Capitalism.' *New Left Review* 146: 53–92.

Jobe, Frank W., Neal ElAttrache, and Ted G. Rand. 1999. *Athletic Forever: The Kerlen–Jobe Orthopaedic Clinic Plan for Lifetime Fitness*: New York: Contemporary.

Johnson, Fenton. 1998. 'Beyond Belief.' *Harper's*, Sept. 1998, 39–54.

Jordan, Tim. 1995. 'Collective Bodies: Raving and the Politics of Gilles Deleuze and Felix Guattari.' *Body and Society* 1 (1): 125–44.

Kafka, Franz. 1961. 'In the Penal Settlement.' In *Metamorphosis and Other Stories*. Harmondsworth: Penguin.

Kant, Immanuel. 1965. *Metaphysical Elements of Justice*. Trans. J. Ladd. Indianapolis: Bobbs-Merrill.

Katzmarzyk, Peter T., Norman Gledhill, and Roy J. Shephard. 2000. 'The Economic Burden of Physical Inactivity in Canada.' *Canadian Medical Association Journal* 163 (11): 1435–40.

Keller, Evelyn Fox. 1989. 'The Gender/Science System: or, Is Sex to Gender As Nature Is to Science?' In N. Tuana, ed., *Feminism and Science*. Bloomington: Indiana University Press.

– 1992. *Secrets of Life, Secrets of Death: Essays on Language, Gender and Science.* New York: Routledge.

Kheel, Marti. 1988. 'Ecofeminism and Deep Ecology?' *Elmwood Newsletter* (winter).

– 1990. 'Ecofeminism and Deep Ecology: Reflections on Identity and Difference.' In I. Diamond and G.F. Orenstein, eds., *Reweaving the World: The Emergence of Ecofeminsm.* San Francisco: Sierra Club Books.

Kickbusch, Ilona. 1994. 'Introduction: Tell Me a Story.' In Pederson, O'Neill, and Rootman 1994.

Kidd, Bruce. 1987. 'Sports and Masculinity.' In M. Kaufman, ed., *Beyond Patriarchy: Essays by Men on Masculinity.* Toronto: Oxford University Press.

Kipnis, Larua. 1993. *Ecstasy Unlimited: On Sex, Capital, Gender, and Aesthetics.* Minneapolis: University of Minnesota Press.

Kirk, David. 1986. 'The Curriculum and Physical Education: Towards a Critical Perspective. Paper read at Commonwealth and International Conference on Sport, Physical Education, Dance, Recreation and Health,' 18–23 July, Glascow.

– 1994. 'Physical Education and Regimes of the Body.' *Australian and New Zealand Journal of Sociology* 30 (2).

Kirk, David, and Barbara Spiller. 1994. 'Schooling the Docile Body: Physical Education, Schooling and the Myth of Oppression.' *Australian Journal of Education* 38 (1): 78–95.

Kirk, David, and Richard Tinning. 1994. 'Embodied Self-identity, Healthy Lifestyles and School Physical Education.' *Sociology of Health and Illness* 16 (5): 600–25.

Kirk, David, and Karen Twigg. 1994. 'Regulating Australian Bodies: Eugenics, Anthropometrics and School Medical Inspection in Victoria, 1900–1940.' *History of Education Review* 23 (1): 19–37.

– 1995. 'Civilizing Australian Bodies: The Games Ethic and Sport in Victorian Government Schools, 1904–1945.' *Sporting Traditions* 11 (2): 3–34.

Krauze, E. 1977. *Power and Illness.* New york: Elsevier.

Krell, David Farrell. 1977a. Introductory comments to Heidegger's essay 'The Question Concerning Technology.' In Krell 1977b.

– ed. *Martin Heidegger: Basic Writings.* New York: Harper and Row.

– 1997. *Architecture: Ecstasies of Space, Time and the Human Body.* Albany: State University of New York Press.

Kristeva, Julia. 1980. 'The Bounded Text.' In L.S. Roudiez, ed., *Desire in Language: A Semiotic Approach to Literature and Art.* New York: Columbia University Press.

- 1982. *Powers of Horror: An Essay on Abjection*. New York: Columbia University Press.

Kuhn, Thomas. 1970. *The Structure of Scientific Revolutions*. Ed. O. Neurath, *International Encyclopedia of Unified Science*. Chicago: Chicago University Press.

Kumar, Shedev. 2000. 'The Truest Test of Faith.' *Globe and Mail*, 24 July 2000, R5.

Laberge, S., and D Sankoff. 1988. 'Physical Activities, Body Habitus, and Lifestyles.' In J. Harvey and H. Cantelon, eds., *Not Just a Game: Essays in Canadian Sports Sociology*. Ottawa: University of Ottawa Press.

Lakka, T.A., J.M. Venalainen, R. Rauramaa, R. Salonen, J. Tuomilehto, and J.T. Salonen. 1994. 'Relation of Leisure-time Physical Activity and Cardiorespiratory Fitness to the Risk of Acute Myocardial Infarction.' *New England Journal of Medicine* 330 (22): 1549–54.

Lalonde, Marc. 1974. *A New Perspective on the Health of Canadians*. Ottawa: Canada Department of Health and Welfare.

Lash, Scott. 1990. *Sociology of Postmodernism*. London: Routledge.

- 1996. 'Postmodern Ethics: The Missing Ground.' *Theory, Culture and Society* 13 (2): 91–104.

Latour, Bruno. 1987. *Science in Action*. Cambridge, Mass.: Harvard University Press.

- 1993. *We Have Never Been Modern*. Trans. C. Porter. Cambridge, Mass.: Harvard University Press.

Latour, Bruno, and Steve Woolgar. 1986. *Laboratory Life: The Construction of Scientific Facts*. Princeton, NJ: Princeton University Press.

Lee, I.M., C.C. Hsieh, and R.S. Paffenbarger, Jr. 1995. 'Exercise Intensity and Longevity in Men: The Harvard Alumni Health Study.' *Journal of the American Medical Association* 273: 1179–1184.

Lee, I.M., and R.S. Paffenbarger, Jr. 2000. 'Associations of Light, Moderate, and Vigorous Intensity Physical Activity with Longevity. The Harvard Alumni Health Study.' *American Journal of Epidemiology* 151 (3): 293–9.

Lee, I.M., R.S. Paffenbarger, Jr, and C.H. Hennekens. 1997. 'Physical Activity, Physical Fitness and Longevity.' *Aging (Milano)* 9 (1–2): 2–11.

Lelwica, Michelle Mary. 1999. *Starving for Salvation: The Spiritual Dimensions of Eating Problems among American Girls and Women*. New York: Oxford University Press.

Lenskyj, Helen. 1992. 'I Am But You Can't Tell.' Paper read to North American Society for the Sociology of Sport, Toledo, Ohio.

Levin, David Michael. 1985. *The Body's Recollection of Being: Phenomenological Psychology and the Deconstruction of Nihilism*. London: Routledge & Kegan Paul.

- 1987a. 'Mudra As Thinking: Developing Our Wisdom-of-Being in Gesture and Movement.' In G. Parkes, ed., *Heidegger and Asian Thought*. Honolulu: University of Hawaii Press.
- ed. 1987b. *Pathologies of the Modern Self: Postmodern Studies on Narcissism, Schizophrenia, and Depression*. New York: New York University Press.

Lingis, Alphonso. 1983. *Excesses: Eros and Culture*. Albany: SUNY Press.
- 1994. *The Community of Those Who Have Nothing In Common*. Bloomington: Indiana University Press.

Llewellyn, John. 1991. *The Middle Voice of Ecological Conscience*. New York: St Martin's Press.
- 1993. *The Song of the Earth*. Bloomington: Indiana University Press.

Lloyd, Moya. 1996. 'Feminism, Aerobics and the Politics of the Body.' *Body and Society* 2 (2): 79–98.

Longino, Helen. 1989. 'Can There Be a Feminist Science?' In N. Tuana, ed., *Feminism and Science*. Bloomington: Indiana University Press.

Lyotard, Jean-Francois. 1984. *The Postmodern Condition: A Report on Knowledge*. Trans. G. Bennington and B. Massumi. Minneapolis: University of Minnesota Press.

McArdle, William R., Frank I. Katch, and Victor L. Katch. 1996. *Exercise Physiology: Energy, Nutrition and Human Performance*. 4th ed. Baltimore: Williams and Wilkins.

MacDonald, Helen. 1985. *Eating for the Health of It: A New Look at Nutrition*. Pridis, Alta.: Austin Books.

MacIntosh, Donald. 1986. 'Physical Education in Higher Education: A Canadian Perspective.' Paper read at Eighth Commonwealth and International Conference on Sport, Physical Education, Dance, Recreation and Health, 18–23 July, at Glasgow.

MacIntosh, Donald, and David Whitson. 1990. *The Game Planners: Transforming Canada's Sport System*. Kingston, Ont.: McGill-Queen's University Press.

McKay, Jim, Jennifer M. Gore, and David Kirk. 1990. 'Beyond the Limits of Technocratic Physical Education.' *Quest* 42 (1): 52–76.

McKeown, T. 1976. *The Role of Medicine: Dream, Mirage, or Nemesis?* London: Nuffield Provincial Hospitals Trust.

MacKinnon, Catherine. 1982. 'Women, Self-possession, and Sport.' In *Feminism Unmodified: Discourse on Life and Law*. Cambridge, Mass.: Harvard University Press.

MacNeill, Margaret. 1994. 'Active Women, Media Representations, and Ideology.' In S. Birrell and C. Cole, eds., *Women, Sport and Culture*. Champaign, Ill.: Human Kinetics.

MacPherson, G., ed. 1992. *Black's Medical Dictionary*. 37th ed. London: A. & C. Black.

Marcuse, Herbert. 1969. *Eros and Civilization*. London: Sphere Books.

Markula, Pirko. 1995. 'Firm But Shapely, Fit But Sexy, Strong But Thin: The Postmodern Aerobicizing of Female Bodies.' *Sociology of Sport Journal* 12 (4).

Martin, Calvin Luther. 1992. *In the Spirit of the Earth: Rethinking History and Time*. Baltimore: Johns Hopkins University Press.

– 1999. *The Way of the Human Being*. New Haven, Conn.: Yale University Press.

Martin, E. 1989. *The Woman in the Body*. Milton Keynes: Open University Press.

Massumi, Brian. 1992. *A User's Guide to Capitalism and Schizophrenia: Deviations from Deleuze and Guattari*. Cambridge, Mass.: MIT Press.

– 1997. 'Realer Than Real: The Similacrum According to Deleuze and Guattari:' http://www.anu.edu.au/HRC/first_and_last/works/realer.htm

Menser, Michael, and Stanley Aronowitz. 1996. ' On Cultural Studies, Science and Technology.' In S. Aronowitz, B. Martinsons, and M. Menser, eds., *Technoscience and Cyberculture*. New York: Routledge.

Merleau-Ponty, Maurice. 1962. *Phenomenology of Perception*. London: Routledge.

– 1968. *The Visible and the Invisible*. Trans. A. Lingis. Evanston, Ill.: Northwestern University Press.

Merton, R., and H. Zuckerman. 1973. 'Institutionalized Patterns of Evaluation in Science.' In N. Storer, ed., *The Sociology of Science*. Chicago: University of Chicago Press.

Messner, Michael. 1992. *Power at Play*. Boston: Beacon.

– 1996. 'Studying Up on Sex.' *Sociology of Sport Journal* 13: 221–37.

Messner, Michael, and Don Sabo, eds. 1990. *Sport, Men and the Gender Order: Critical Feminist Perspectives*. Champaign, Ill.: Human Kinetics.

– 1994. *Sex, Violence and Power in Sports: Rethinking Masculinity*. Freedom, Calif.: Crossing Press.

Micheli, Lyle J., and Mark D. Jenkins. 1995. *The Sports Medicine Bible: Prevent, Detect, and Treat Your Sports Injuries through the Latest Medical Techniques*. New York: HarperCollins.

Miles, Steven. 1998. *Consumerism – As a Way of Life*. London: Sage.

Miller, Toby. 1993. *The Well-tempered Self: Citizenship, Culture and the Postmodern Subject*. Baltimore: Johns Hopkins University Press.

Moi, Tori. 2000. *What Is a Woman? And Other Essays*. Oxford: Oxford University Press.

Monk, W.H. 1933. 'Eventide.' In *The English Hymnal*. Oxford: Oxford University Press.

Moore, Pamela, ed. 1997. *Building Bodies*. New Brunswick, NJ: Rutgers University Press.

Morris, J.N., D.G. Clayton, M.G. Everitt, A.M. Semmence, and E.H. Burgess. 1990. 'Exercise in Leisure Time: Coronary Attack and Death Rates.' *British Heart Journal* 63 (6): 325–34.

Morris, J.N., M.G. Everitt, R. Pollard, S.P. Chave, and A.M. Semmence. 1980. 'Vigorous Exercise in Leisure-Time: Protection against Coronary Heart Disease.' *Lancet* 2 (8206): 1207–10.

Morrison, Paul. 1996. *The Poetics of Fascism: Ezra Pound, T.S. Eliot, Paul de Man.* New York: Oxford University Press.

Morton, Donald, ed. 1996. *The Material Queer: A LesBiGay Studies Reader.* Boulder, Col.: Westview.

Mrozek, Donald J. 1987. 'The Scientific Quest for Physical Education and the Persistent Appeal of Quackery.' *Journal of Sport History* 14 (1): 76–86.

Nancy, Jean-Luc. 1993. *The Experience of Freedom.* Trans. B. McDonald. Stanford, Calif.: Stanford University Press.

Nelson, Richard. 1994. 'Biomechanics in Exercise Science and Sports Medicine.' In ACSM 1994.

Newton, Isaac. 1934. *Philosophiae Naturalis Principia Mathematica.* Trans. A. Motte, ed. F. Cajavi. Cambridge: Cambridge University Press.

Nietzsche, Friedrich. 1956. *The Genealogy of Morals.* In *The Birth of Tragedy and The Genealogy of Morals.* Garden City, NY: Doubleday.

Noble, David. 1992. *A World without Women: The Christian Clerical Tradition of Western Science.* New York: Oxford University Press.

Ontario. 1974. *Report of the Health Planning Task Force.* Toronto: Ministry of Health.

Paffenbarger, R.S., Jr, J.B. Kampert, and I.M. Lee. 1997. 'Physical Activity and Health of College Men: Longitudinal Observations.' *International Journal of Sports Medicine* 18 (supp. 3): S200–3.

Parkes, Graham, ed. 1987. *Heidegger and Asian Thought.* Honolulu: University of Hawaii Press.

Pate, R.R., M. Pratt, S.N. Blair, W.L. Haskell, C.A. Macera, C. Bouchard, D. Buchner, W. Ettinger, G.W. Heath, A.C. King, et al. 1995. 'Physical Activity and Public Health. A Recommendation from the Centers for Disease Control and Prevention and the American College of Sports Medicine' (see comments). *Journal of the American Medical Association* 273 (5): 402–7.

Pederson, Ann, Michel O'Neill, and Irving Rootman. 1994. *Health Promotion in Canada: Provincial, National and International Perspectives.* Toronto: W.B. Saunders.

Peterson, Alan. 1997. 'Risk, Governance and the New Public Health.' In Peterson and Bunton 1997.

Peterson, Alan, and Robin Bunton, eds. 1997. *Foucault, Health and Medicine.* London: Routledge.

Phelan, Shane. 1994. *Getting Specific: Postmodern Lesbian Politics*. Minneapolis: University of Minnesota Press.

Phillips, Bill. 1997. *Sports Supplement Review: Build Muscle! Lose Fat! What Works? What Doesn't?* Golden, Col.: Mile High Publishing.

Pickering, Andrew. 1992. 'From Science As Knowledge to Science As Practice.' In A. Pickering, ed., *Science As Practice and Culture*. Chicago: University of Chicago Press.

– 1995. *The Mangle of Practice: Time, Agency and Science*. Chicago: University of Chicago Press.

Pinder, Lavada. 1988. 'From *A New Perspective* to the *Framework*.' *Health Promotion, an International Journal* 3 (2): 205–12.

– 1994. 'The Federal Role in Health Promotion: Art of the Possible.' In Pederson, O'Neill, and Rootman 1994.

Polanyi, John. 2000. 'Quest for Truly Social Science.' *Globe and Mail*, 29 April 2000, A 19.

Powels, J. 1973. 'On the Limitations of Modern Medicine.' *Science, Medicine, and Man* 1 (1): 1–30.

Probyn, Elspeth. 1995. 'Queer Belongings: The Politics of Departure.' In Grosz and Probyn 1995.

Pronger, Brian. 1990a. *The Arena of Masculinity: Sports, Homosexuality and the Meaning of Sex*. 1st ed. New York: St Martin's Press.

– 1990b. 'Being Loves to Hide Itself: Reflections on the Psychology of Ereignis.' Paper read to Society for Phenomenology and the Human Sciences, 12 Oct., Villanova.

– 1990c. 'Gay Jocks: A Phenomenology of Gay Men in Athletics.' In Messner and Sabo 1990. Champaign, Ill.: Human Kinetics.

– 1991a. 'Disclosures of Human Being: A New Terrain for the Psychology of Physical Activity.' Master of science thesis, University of Toronto, Toronto.

– 1991b. 'Muscling In: Pleasure in the Embodiment of Denial.' Paper read to North American Society for the Sociology of Sport, 9 Nov., Milwaukee, Wisc.

– 1992a. *The Arena of Masculinity: Sports, Homosexuality and the Meaning of Sex*. 2nd ed. Toronto: University of Toronto Press.

– 1992b. 'Resisting Pleasure, Pleasure Resisting.' Paper read to North American Society for the Sociology of Sport, 7 Nov., Toledo, Ohio.

– 1994. 'Body Territory: Sport and the Art of Non-Fascist Living.' Paper read to North American Society for the Sociology of Sport, 12 Nov., Savannah, Ga.

– 1995a. 'Eros, Thanatos: The Emerging Body in a Postmodern Psychology of Science.' In B. Babich, D. Bergoffen, and S. Glynn, eds., *Continental and Postmodern Perspectives in the Philosophy of Science*. Aldershot: Avebury.

– 1995b. 'Rendering the Body: The Implicit Lessons of Gross Anatomy.' *Quest* 47 (4): 1–20.
– 1996. 'Political Power in the Science of Physical Fitness.' PhD thesis, Graduate Department of Community Health, University of Toronto.
– 1998a. 'On Your Knees: Carnal Knowledge, Masculine Dissolution, Doing Feminism.' In T. Digby, ed., *Men Doing Feminism*. New York: Routledge.
– 1998b. 'Post-Sport: Transgressing Boundaries in Physical Culture.' In G. Rail, ed., *Sport and Postmodern Times: Culture, Gender, Sexuality, the Body and Sport*. Buffalo: SUNY Press.
– 1999a. 'Fear and Trembling: Homophobia in Men's Sport.' In P. White and K. Young, eds., *Sport and Gender in Canada*. Toronto: Oxford University Press.
– 1999b. 'Outta My Endzone: Sport and the Territorial Anus.' *Journal of Sport and Social Issues* 23 (4): 373–89.
– 2000. 'Homosexuality and Sport: Who's Winning?' In J. McKay, M. Messner, and D. Sabo, eds., *Masculinities and Sport*. London: Sage.
Radloff, Bernhard. 1993. 'Text.' In I. Makaryk, ed., *Encyclopedia of Contemporary Literary Theory: Approaches, Scholars, Terms*. Toronto: University of Toronto Press.
Readings, Bill, and Bennet Schaber, eds. 1993. *Postmodernism across the Ages*. Syracuse, NY: Syracuse University Press.
Rilke, Rainer Maria. 1989. *The Selected Poetry of Rainer Maria Rilke*. Trans. S. Mitchell. New York: Vintage.
– 1996. 'Death.' In *Uncollected Poems of Rainer Maria Rilke*. New York: North Point Press, Farrar, Straus and Giroux.
Robbe-Grillet, Alain. 1965. *For a New Novel*. Trans. R. Howard. New York: Grove.
Rockefeller, Steven C. 1992. 'Faith and Community in an Ecological Age.' In S.C. Rockefeller and J.C. Elder, ed., *Spirit and Nature: Why the Environment Is a Religious Issue*. Boston: Beacon Press.
Rootman, Irving, and Michel O'Neill. 1994. 'Developing Knowledge for Health Promotion.' In Pederson, O'Neill, and Rootman 1994.
Rootman, Irving, and John Raeburn. 1994. 'The Concept of Health.' In Pederson, O'Neill, and Rootman 1994.
Rosenthal, Michael. 1992. 'What Was Postmodernism?' *Socialist Review*: 83–105.
Rosser, Sue. 1990. *Female-friendly Science: Applying Women's Studies Methods and Theories to Attract Students*. New York: Pergamon Press.
Rouse, Joseph. 1987. *Knowledge and Power: Toward a Political Philosophy of Science*. Ithaca, NY: Cornell University Press.
Rushdie, Salman. 1999. *The Ground beneath Her Feet*. Toronto: Knopf.

Said, Edward. 1978 (1994). *Orientalism*. New York: Vintage.

– 1993. *Culture and Imperialism*. New York: Knopf.

Schell, Johnathan. 2000. 'The Unfinished Twentieth Century: What We Have Forgotten about Nuclear Weapons.' *Harpers*, Jan. 2000, 41–56.

Schlosberg, Suzanne, and Liz Neporent. 1996. *Fitness for Dummies*. Foster City, Calif.: IDG Books Worldwide.

Seem, Mark. 1983. 'Introduction.' In Deleuze and Guattari 1983.

Seid, Roberta Pollack. 1989. *Never Too Thin: Why Women Are at War with Their Bodies*. New York: Prentice Hall.

Seidman, Steven. 1993. 'Identity Politics in a "Postmodern" Gay Culture: Some Historical and Conceptual Notes.' In Warner 1993.

Sesso, H.D., R.S. Paffenbarger, Jr, and I.M. Lee. 2000. 'Physical Activity and Coronary Heart Disease in Men: The Harvard Alumni Health Study.' *Circulation (Online)* 102 (9): 975–80.

Shangold, M.M. 1988. *Women and Exercise: Physiology and Sports Medicine*. 2nd ed. Philadelphia: F.A. Davis.

Shapin, Steven. 1994. *A Social History of Truth: Civility and Science in Seventeenth-Century England*. Chicago: University of Chicago Press.

Shapin, Steven, and Simon Schaffer. 1985. *Leviathan and the Air Pump: Hobbes, Boyle, and the Experimental Life*. Princeton, NJ: Princeton University Press.

Sheehan, Thomas. 1981. 'On Movement and the Destruction of Ontology.' *Monist* 64: 534–42.

– 1983. 'On the Way to *Ereignis*: Heidegger's Interpretation of *Physis*.' In H. Silverman, J. Sallis, and T. Seebohm, eds., *Continental Philosophy in America*. Pittsburgh: Duquesne University Press.

Sheng-yen. 1999. *Complete Enlightenment: Zen Comments on the Sutra of Complete Enlightenment*. Boston: Shambhala.

Shephard, Roy J. 1986a. *Economic Benefits of Enhanced Fitness*. Champaign, Ill.: Human Kinetics.

– 1986b. *Fitness and Health in Industry*. Basel: Karger.

– 1994. 'Physical Activity, Fitness, and Health: The Current Consensus.' *Quest* 47 (3): 288–303.

Shilling, Chris. 1993. *The Body and Social Theory*. London: Sage.

Silverman, Hugh, ed. 1989. *Derrida and Deconstruction*. New York: Routledge.

Simpson, Mark, ed. 1996. *Anti-Gay*. London: Cassell.

Sinfield, Alan. 1994. *Cultural Politics – Queer Reading*. Philadelphia: University of Pennsylvania Press.

Skinner, Harvey A. 1994a. 'Computerized Lifestyle Assessment.' Toronto: Multi-Health Systems.

- 1994b. *Computerized Lifestyle Assessment: User Manual*. Toronto: Multi-Health Systems.

Slattery, M.L., D.R. Jacobs, Jr, and M.Z. Nichaman. 1989. 'Leisure Time Physical Activity and Coronary Heart Disease Death: The US Railroad Study.' *Circulation* 79: 304–11.

Smart, Barry. 1990. 'Modernity, Postmodernity and the Present.' In Bryan Turner, ed., 1990.

Sparks, Robert. 1990. 'Social Practice, the Bodily Professions and the State.' *Sociology of Sport Journal* 7 (1): 72–82.

Spitzack, Carole. 1990. *Confessing Excess: Women and the Politics of Body Reduction*. Albany: State University of New York Press.

Spivak, Gayatri Chakravorty. 1995. 'Can the Subaltern Speak?' In Ashcroft, Griffiths, and Tiffin 1995.

Spretnak, Charelen. 1990. 'Ecofeminism: Our Roots Are Flowering.' In I. Diamond and G.F. Orenstein, eds., *Reweaving the World: The Emergence of Ecofeminism*. San Francisco: Sierra Club Books.

Stambaugh, Joan. 1990. *Impermanence Is Buddha-nature: Dogen's Understanding of Temporality*. Honolulu: University of Hawaii Press.

Standing Committee on Health and Welfare, Social Affairs, Seniors and the Status of Women. 1991. *The War against Women*. Ottawa: Government of Canada.

Stein, Edward. 1992. *Forms of Desire: Sexual Orientation and the Social Constructionist Controversy*. New York: Routledge.

Stein, H. 1982. 'Neo-Darwinism and Survival through Fitness in Reagan's America.' *Journal of Psychohistory* 10 (fall): 163–87.

Stivale, Charles. 1998. *The Two-fold Thought of Deleuze and Guattari*. New York: Guilford Press.

Surin, Kenneth. 1998. 'Liberation.' In M. Taylor, ed., *Critical Terms for Religious Studies*. Chicago: University of Chicago Press.

Taylor, Mark. 1984. *Erring: A Postmodern A/theology*. Chicago: University of Chicago Press.

- 1987. *Altarity*. Chicago: University of Chicago Press.

- 1990. *Tears*. Albany: SUNY Press.

Tough, Paul. 1996. 'Does America Still Work? On the Turbulent Energies of the New Capitalism.' *Harpers*, May, 35–47.

Turner, Bryan. 1984. *The Body and Society*. Oxford: Basil Blackwell.

- ed. 1990. *Theories of Modernity and Postmodernity*. London: Sage.

- 1991. 'Recent Developments in the Theory of the Body.' In Featherstone, Hepworth, and Turner 1991.

- 1992. *Regulating Bodies: Essays in Medical Sociology*. New York: Routledge.
- 1997. 'The Body in Western Society: Social Theory and Its Perspectives.' In S. Coakley, ed., *Religion and the Body*. Cambridge: Cambridge University Press.

Turner, Frederick. 1991. *Beauty: The Value of Values*. Charlottesville: University of Virginia.

U.S. Department of Health and Human Services. 1996. *Physical Activity and Health: A Report of the Surgeon General*. Atlanta, Ga.: U.S. Department of Health and Human Services, Centers for Disease Control and Prevention, National Center for Chronic Disease Prevention and Health Promotion.

Vertinsky, Patricia. 1991. 'Old Age, Gender and Physical Activity: The Biomedicalization of Aging.' *Journal of Sport History* 18 (1): 64–80.
- 1992. 'Exercise, Physical Capability and the Eternally Wounded Woman in Late Nineteenth-century North America.' In J. Berryman and R. Park, eds., *Sport and Exercise Science: Essays in the History of Sports Medicine*. Chicago: University of Illinois Press.
- 1995. 'The "Racial" Body and the Anatomy of Difference: Anti-semitism, Physical Culture, and the Jew's Foot.' *Sport Science Review* 4 (1): 38–59.

Warner, Michael, ed. 1993. *Fear of a Queer Planet: Queer Politics and Social Theory*. Minneapolis: University of Minnesota Press.

Wheeler, John Archibald. 1982. 'Bohr, Enstein, and the Strange Lesson of the Quantum.' In R.Q. Elvee, ed., *Mind in Nature: Nobel Conference XVII*. New York: Harper and Row.

Whitson, David. 1990. 'Sport in the Social Construction of Masculinity.' In Messner and Sabo 1990.
- 1994. 'The Embodiment of Gender: Discipline, Domination, and Empowerment.' In S. Birrell and C.L. Cole, eds., *Women, Sport, and Culture*. Champaign, Ill.: Human Kinetics.

Whitson, David, and Donald MacIntosh. 1990. 'The Scientization of Physical Education: Discourses of Performance.' *Quest* 42 (1): 40–51.

Williams, Raymond. 1977. *Marxism and Literature*. London: Oxford University Press.
- 1980. *Problems in Materialism and Culture*. London: Verso.

Wolf, Naomi. 1990. *The Beauty Myth*. London: Vintage.

World Health Organization (WHO). 1984. *Health Promotion: A Discussion Document on the Concept and Principles*. Copenhagen: World Health Organization, Regional Office for Europe.
- 1986. *Ottawa Charter for Health Promotion*. Ottawa: Canadian Public Health Association.

Zimmerman, Michael. 1987. Feminism, Deep Ecology and Environmental Ethics. *Environmental Ethics* 9 (1).

Index